A Neurosurgeon's Notebook

One man's way of trying to avoid trouble

CHRIS ADAMS

MA, MChir, FRCS
Consultant Neurosurgeon, The Radcliffe Infirmary, Oxford
Lecturer in Neurosurgery, The University of Oxford
Fellow, Green College, Oxford
Member of the American Association of Neurological Surgeons

FOREWORD BY
MICHAEL APUZZO

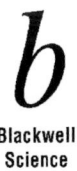

Blackwell
Science

To my trainees for their stimulation,
motivation and friendship

© 1998 by C. Adams and
Blackwell Science Ltd
Editorial Offices:
Osney Mead, Oxford OX2 0EL
25 John Street, London WC1N 2BL
23 Ainslie Place, Edinburgh EH3 6AJ
350 Main Street, Malden
    MA 02148 5018, USA
54 University Street, Carlton
    Victoria 3053, Australia
10, rue Casimir Delavigne
    75006 Paris, France

Other Editorial Offices:
Blackwell Wissenschafts-Verlag GmbH
Kurfürstendamm 57
10707 Berlin, Germany

Blackwell Science KK
MG Kodenmacho Building
7–10 Kodenmacho Nihombashi
Chuo-ku, Tokyo 104, Japan

The right of the Author to be
identified as the Author of this Work
has been asserted in accordance
with the Copyright, Designs and
Patents Act 1988.

First published 1998
Reprinted 1999 (twice)

Set by Excel Typesetters Co., Hong Kong
Printed and bound in Great Britain
at the Alden Press Ltd.,
Oxford and Northampton

DISTRIBUTORS

Marston Book Services Ltd
PO Box 269
Abingdon, Oxon OX14 4YN
(*Orders*: Tel: 01235 465500
          Fax: 01235 465555)

USA
Blackwell Science, Inc.
Commerce Place
350 Main Street
Malden, MA 02148 5018
(*Orders*: Tel: 800 759 6102
                781 388 8250
          Fax: 781 388 8255)

Canada
Login Brothers Book Company
324 Saulteaux Crescent
Winnipeg, Manitoba R3J 3T2
(*Orders*: Tel: 204 837-2987)

Australia
Blackwell Science Pty Ltd
54 University Street
Carlton, Victoria 3053
(*Orders*: Tel: 3 9347 0300
          Fax: 3 9347 5001)

A catalogue record for this title
is available from the British Library
and the Library of Congress

ISBN 0-632-05154-X

For further information on
Blackwell Science, visit our website:
www.blackwell-science.com

The Blackwell Science logo is a
trade mark of Blackwell Science Ltd,
registered at the United Kingdom
Trade Marks Registry

Contents

Foreword

MICHAEL L. J. APUZZO, MD

Edwin M. Todd/Trent H. Wells, Jr., Professor of Neurological Surgery and Radiation Oncology, Biology and Physics, University of Southern California School of Medicine, Los Angeles, California, USA
Editor-in-Chief, Neurosurgery
President, US Congress of Neurological Surgeons

Summa cum laude

Embarking upon a career in neurological surgery carries a charge to master, and requires an effort to take control of what is an immense, ever-changing and rapidly evolving body of knowledge. It represents an unusually challenging goal which requires strength of body, mind and spirit. It is without doubt a laudable but simultaneously a foolhardy ambition, as complete mastery is a lifelong quixotic quest but one which attracts the brightest and the most passionate, but often those who are naïve to the enormity of the challenge and task.

Confronted by these realities, it would seem that the embryonic student would benefit from a succinct and rudimentary statement of quintessential foundations from a scholarly master in the field—a statement of fundamental principles, important nuances and key attitudes to serve as groundwork and compass in a complex and ever-changing field—a statement of experience made with an eye to the element of art, humanity and persona of the discipline.

This perspective evolves from lessons that are hard-learned and demand the utmost attention and absolute digestion of the neophyte.

Chris Adams has produced a unique and important product presenting and distilling to their essence a multiplicity of essential points, gleaned and intelligently perceived during an intense and challenging, practical and academic neurosurgical career. These are points which serve as a foundation for the newly baptized student and a compass for the experienced journeyman or master. Such a handbook in size, directive and perspective has not been available to the young neurosurgeon in the past. It is long overdue and will be as essential to them as their reflex hammer or imaging device.

Bravo, Mr Adams! Bravo, bravissimo!

Preface

I vowed never to write a book on neurosurgery for several reasons, but mainly to avoid replicating what has been well written already. Pressure, mainly from my residents (trainees), has resulted in producing this notebook. In one sense this has taken a lifetime to write and it certainly represents 30 years of neurosurgical experience, often bitter experience. Inevitably one does learn from experience, especially from the more bitter variety, and I had to agree with my younger colleagues that it was a pity not to try to attempt to pass on some of these lessons. I have actually kept a notebook for the 30 years I have been doing neurosurgery. I advise trainees to do the same and to obtain their own notebook to jot down ideas, tips and hints, as well as the way they see things done, otherwise they will forget. Even better is to also keep a disaster book to record one's own disasters! All too easily we remember our triumphs but our disasters quickly slip from our consciousness. It would be better if it was the reverse but we are human and share these attributes with other members of the human race.

Some aspects of this book have their genesis in the teaching of trainees. Certain aspects of anatomy cause difficulty for them (and for myself) and so these areas are emphasized. Other aspects concern surgical judgement and the art and philosophy rather than the science of neurosurgery, while Chapter 9 concentrates on technical tips.

Surgical judgement, both clinical and operative, is crucial to the successful performance of neurosurgery. However skilful the surgeon, if he (and increasingly and rightly, she) does the wrong operation at the wrong time, then the patient is not helped or is even harmed. Much of neurosurgery also entails avoiding dangers and all of us have to tread the tortuous and difficult road passing between, doing our best for the patient, yet avoiding harm. To put it in another way, my assistant may on occasions hear me mutter in the operating theatre 'luck favours the bold'. Yet on other occasions 'discretion is the better part of valour'. Yet how do you practise (and teach) judicious boldness and discretion? No one has written a book on this aspect of neuro-surgery and in a sense this is an attempt. Much of this is passed on by word of mouth but hopefully it might prove useful to try to write about it.

In producing this notebook I am not in any way trying to cover all 'neurosurgery'. Indeed, I have rejected writing about aspects well emphasized in standard textbooks. Of course pearls of wisdom are already available in these large multi-author books. These pearls may be difficult to find amongst the huge amount of factual information. In producing my own 'neurosurgical notebook' I am, of course, describing just one man's way of doing things and as my admirable friend the late Charlie Drake said, 'there are many ways to skin a cat'. This is merely my particular method of skinning the neurosurgical cat. By the way, why is Charles Drake so admirable? Mainly because he was one of the few neurosurgeons who went around the world talking about difficulties and complications, rather than his (many) successes. I hope there will be more like him.

This leads me to an early plug for *skepticos*, Greek for scepticism. This is a vital attribute to acquire as early as possible in one's career. Do not believe all you hear or read. Do not believe the contents of this book, but at least think about them. Do not believe the world famous neurosurgeon's slides of an amazing operation. How was the patient? Who assessed him or her? What did the relatives think of the operation? For every wonderful result, how many disasters have been quietly forgotten? Do not believe the scan report, go and look at the scan and work it out for yourself. Do not necessarily believe the latest theory. Does it fit the facts as you find them? Scepticism is a wonderful tool for preserving your own professional reputation, as well as preserving your patients, quite apart from being the motivating force for advancing knowledge.

Perhaps the most important principle is the KISS principle. Ever since hearing a lawyer extolling the virtues of people adhering rigidly to their principles ('it is good for business, makes people litigate'), I have avoided if possible, having any principles at all. Rules yes, principles no. One can always have an exception to a rule to prove the rule. However, one principle I have been forced to maintain, is the KISS principle: 'keep it simple and safe'. Why? Simplicity is actually the external appearance of clarity of thought. If one can make a problem simple, to a patient or a trainee, it means that the neurosurgeon has clarified his or her own thoughts. This in turn is perhaps the greatest factor in engendering confidence in the patient. A 'simple' operation, done quickly yet unhurriedly, reflects clarity of thought and deed by the surgeon. My advice is therefore concentrate on the KISS principle; and avoid the KICK principle ('keep it complicated and knotty'). It never ceases to amaze me how some surgeons embrace the KICK principle, perhaps feeling this enhances their own uniqueness.

It is with considerable humility that I offer my small notebook. I do not know if I have succeeded, even partially, but if I have provoked surgeons to think and ponder, if only to reject rather than to accept, then I will be content. The bare bones of what I have tried to record will not date and should be as relevant today as they were 100 years ago and will be in 100 years' time. This notebook is intended to be your notebook, and space is provided for you to note the things that interest, puzzle or intrigue. It is a book I hope you will keep in your desk drawer throughout your career to add to and improve upon these skeletal notes I have provided; much of what I have written concerns an attitude and an approach, and for that reason alone this small notebook may be of use to a wider audience than just neurosurgeons.

What then, in essence, is this book about? It is my way of avoiding getting into trouble as much as possible. Who then is this book for? For anyone particularly interested in avoiding getting into trouble! It is not just for trainees but also for trained neurosurgeons who have embarked on their professional careers. Some aspects of surgery discussed in this notebook are very basic (but very important) while some quite sophisticated areas are also addressed. Whoever you are and at whatever stage you are at, I hope you enjoy and profit from reading this small notebook. As I have said, I hope it will become your notebook and perhaps you can even jot down your disasters at the back! I wish you luck. See Rule 16.

Acknowledgements

To my trainees for their stimulation, motivation and friendship. My thanks to Professor Andrew Kaye for reading the manuscript and making valuable suggestions. To my secretary Mrs Cathie Theodorou for finding time to type (and retype) this book amongst all the many other things she has to do. To Dr Jean Millar FRCA for allowing me to use (her) Table 9. To Professor Mike Apuzzo for generously agreeing to write the Foreword. To Mrs Angela Walters whose generous donation defrayed the costs of publication of this book.

chapter one

Rules for a happy and trouble-free neurosurgical life!

About 100 years ago, it was common for authors to produce small books of 'rules' for various aspects of life. This didactic approach has rather diminished with the fashion for liberalism and the reluctance of the older generation to tell the younger generation anything. The car sticker 'go out and get a job now that you are 18 and know everything' also reflects the confidence of youth and their reluctance to accept advice. Yet in my experience, neurosurgical trainees are eager for rules, even though these rules are there to be broken occasionally! I record them here in the hope that they might amuse or even stimulate you, and they might even keep you out of trouble!

1   Embrace the KISS principle: 'Keep it simple and safe'.
2   Avoid the KICK principle: 'Keep it complicated and knotty'.
3   Be *sceptical*.
4   Do not operate on scans, but on patients (for surgeons).
5   Do not operate on blood vessels but on people (for interventional neuroradiologists and vascular neurosurgeons).
6   Luck favours the bold.
7   Discretion is the better part of valour.
8   Taking a history is the most difficult and most important 'art' in neurosurgery.
9   Always see the patient and remind oneself of the salient facts immediately before the operation, as well as encouraging the patient. 'A little touch of Harry in the night'.
10   Always have the X-rays and scans in the operating theatre.
11   The operations that go wrong are the 'simple ones' that you haven't thought about.
12   Time taken to position the patient on the operating table is time well spent.
13   The most difficult thing to learn is when to stop an operation.

14   The Laws of Physics a surgeon needs are firstly, light travels in straight lines and so do not bend retractors. Keeping the retractor blade straight avoids brain damage. The second is that water runs downhill, therefore first look for bleeders superficially and then work deeper.

15   Keep a personal 'disaster' book. Write down your disasters and think about them. Doctors have an amazing ability, like fishermen, horse punters and stock-market investors, to forget their failures and only remember their successes. In other words, only make a particular mistake once!

16   A happy surgeon is a 'lucky surgeon'. Actually I believe, a comfortable, stress-free surgeon makes better decisions and operates better than the tense, stressed surgeon.

17   Good judgement and therefore good decisions depend on attention to detail and clear thinking (see Rule 1).

chapter two

Anatomy

The best surgeons are usually the best anatomists; the wondrous electronic aids such as magnetic resonance imaging (MRI) scans and operating arm systems may tempt trainees into believing the age of anatomy has passed. This would be a serious mistake. Indeed, the more procedures we are able to do, the more detailed anatomy we are required to learn. My experience of teaching trainees has shown that there are particular areas of anatomy that are difficult to acquire. This is usually the skull base area, and over the years I have devised a series of simplified diagrams to aid the trainee in having at least a 'ground map' on which to base his or her anatomical knowledge. Detail and accuracy will be acquired later but at least a simplified diagram can form the foundation, especially if associated with examining the spine and skull again and again and yet again! I never fail to be amazed at how much more anatomy I learn year after year! This chapter is essentially a series of diagrams for you to learn, and makes no attempt to teach you detailed anatomy. You will have to do that yourself armed with the bones and a textbook of anatomy, or even better, a cadaver.

The skull base

Adams' grid

Figure 1 is known by my trainees as the 'Adams' grid'. It is composed of four vertical and four horizontal lines. It is in fact accurate in the two planes shown. However, the horizontal 'external auditory meatal line' has four different levels in the third dimension, as shown in Figure 2. An ability to memorize this grid is essential for the performance of skull base surgery. For instance, the 'antero-lateral' approach to the jugular foramen or foramen magnum entails removal of the bone in the order shown in the 'mastoid horizontal line', i.e. mastoid process, digastric groove, jugular

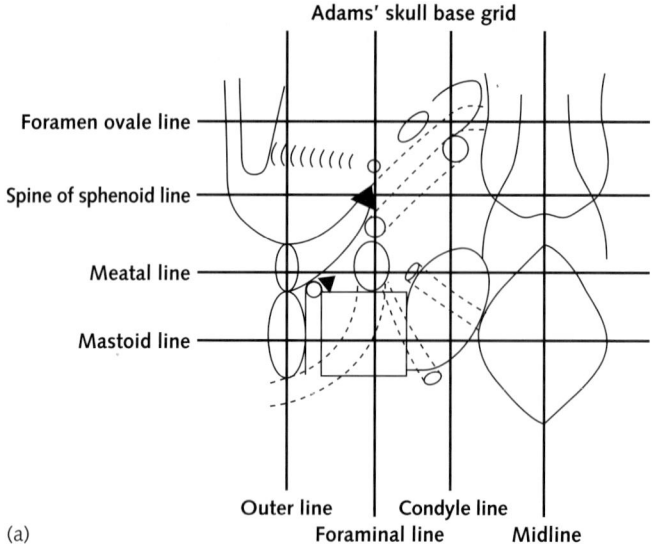

(a)

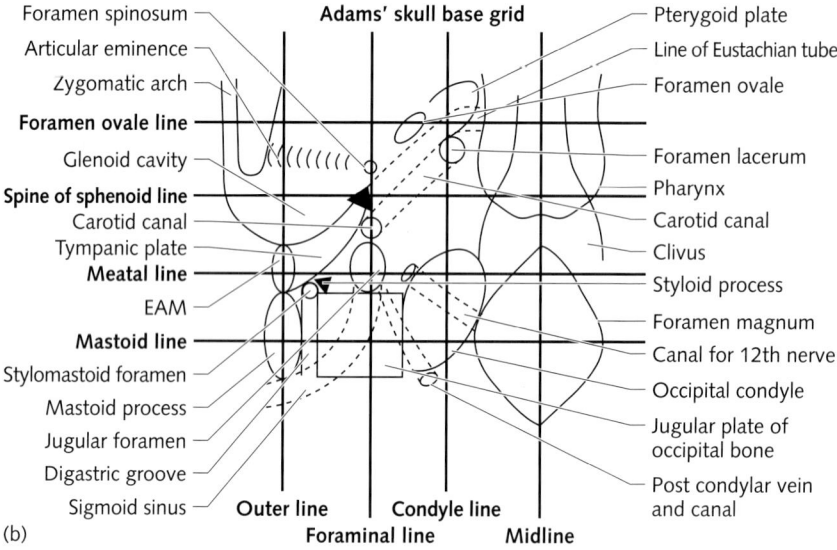

(b)

Fig. 1 (a) 'Adams' grid' of the skull base. (b) The grid labelled. EAM, external auditory meatus.

process of the occipital bone (to which the rectus capitis lateralis muscle is attached), sigmoid sinus and finally the posterior half of the condyle, with of course the surgeon coming into contact with the posterior condylar emissary vein.

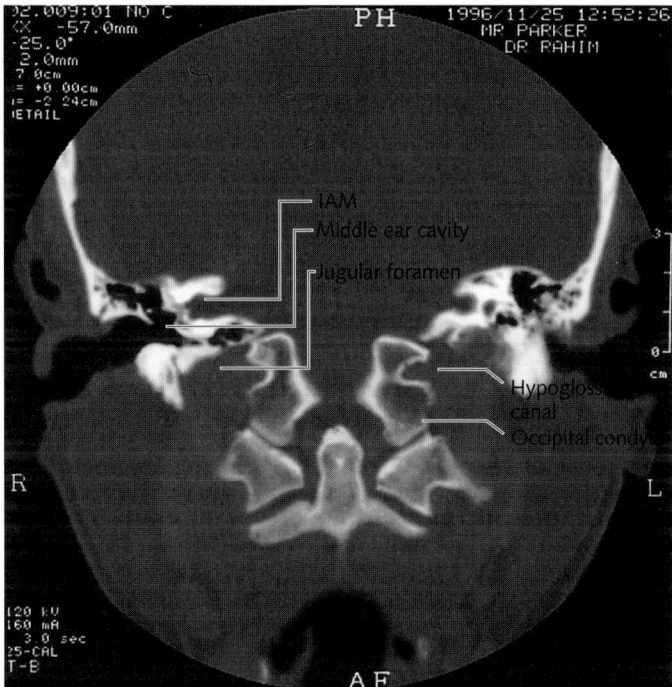

Fig. 2   Four levels of the 'external auditory meatal line'. A coronal bone window CT scan through the EAM to show, on the right, from above down the internal auditory meatus (IAM), the middle ear cavity, the jugular foramen and the occipital condyle. Note the glomus jugulare tumour eroding the left petrous bone in the vicinity of the jugular foramen.

Suboccipital region

Figure 3 diagramatically shows the muscles of the occipital and suboccipital region, the details of which are in my experience often not known. Coupled with this, the trainee should know the 'three curves' of the vertebral artery as it passes from the lower border of C3 to enter the dura at the foramen magnum (Figure 4). Reflecting on the remarkably curvaceous course, one must conclude that this tortuosity is concerned with maintaining blood flow with extreme positions of the head in relation to the neck.

The external meatal line is of particular relevance to the surgery of glomus jugulare tumours. The most important landmark is perhaps the spine of the sphenoid. Whenever one hears mention of that structure, one should immediately say 'carotid canal, Eustachian tube and foramen spinosum', for these three 'holes' are clustered around the spine of the sphenoid. The tympanic plate, forming the antero-inferior component of the bony meatus and middle ear, is triangular in shape and tapers down to an acute angle at the spine of the sphenoid forming the posterior half of the glenoid cavity. To expose the vertical component of the intrapetrous internal carotid artery, it is necessary to dislocate the head of the mandible from the glenoid cavity then drill away the tympanic plate protecting the carotid artery. Knowledge of the grid will help one realize that the Eustachian tube crosses the carotid artery laterally as the tube gently descends to pierce the nasopharyngeal mucosa adjacent to the medial pterygoid plate, while the carotid artery in its horizontal course gently ascends to enter the cavernous sinus. The spine of the sphenoid can be seen on a 'bone window' computed tomography (CT) scan and in my experience is a wonderfully useful landmark. Running above the Eustachian tube is the greater superficial petrosal nerve aiming for the foramen lacerum, being just in front of the horizontal component of the carotid artery. Both these structures cross the foramen lacerum, although the foramen itself is unique in that nothing of note passes through it. The greater superficial petrosal nerve is the landmark to show the surgeon the carotid canal during the subtemporal approach to the skull base. The line drawn from the foramen spinosum to the foramen ovale makes the third

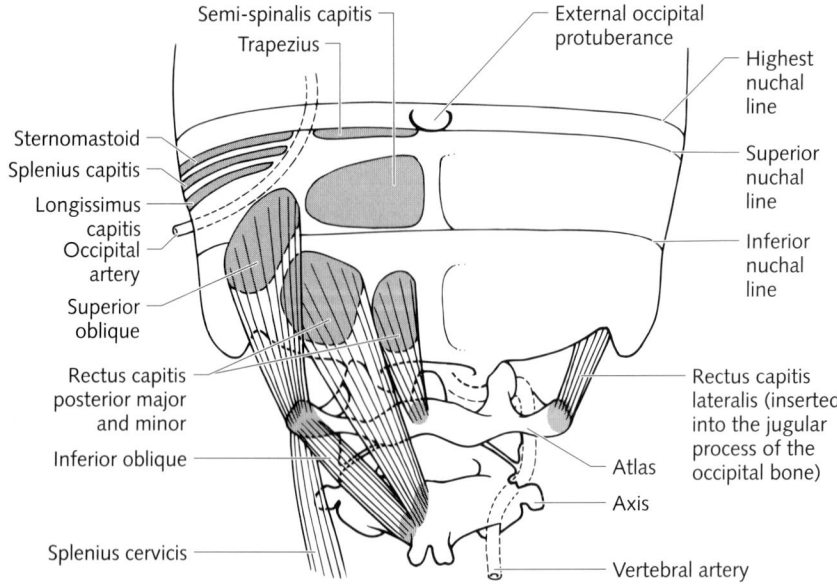

(a)

Fig. 3 (a) Diagram to show the muscles of the suboccipital area. (*Continued*)

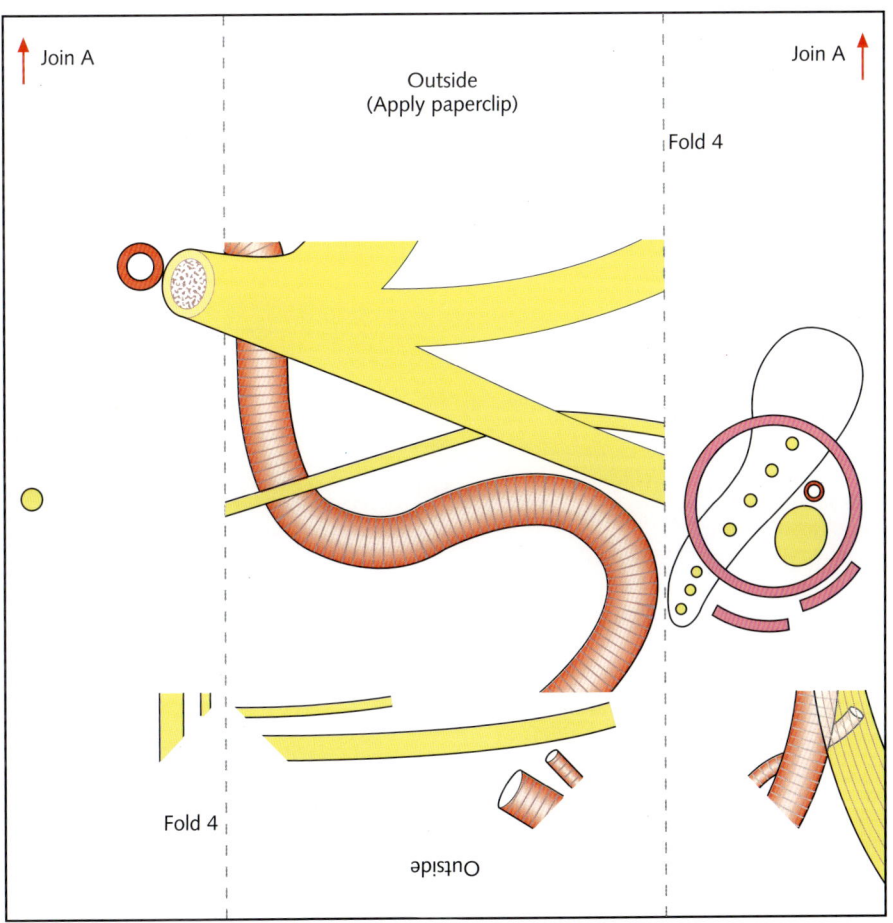

Join A

Outside
(Apply paperclip)

Fold 4

Join A

Fold 4

Outside

Plate 1 Origami of the cavernous sinus. Cut along outside lines, and fold as instructed.

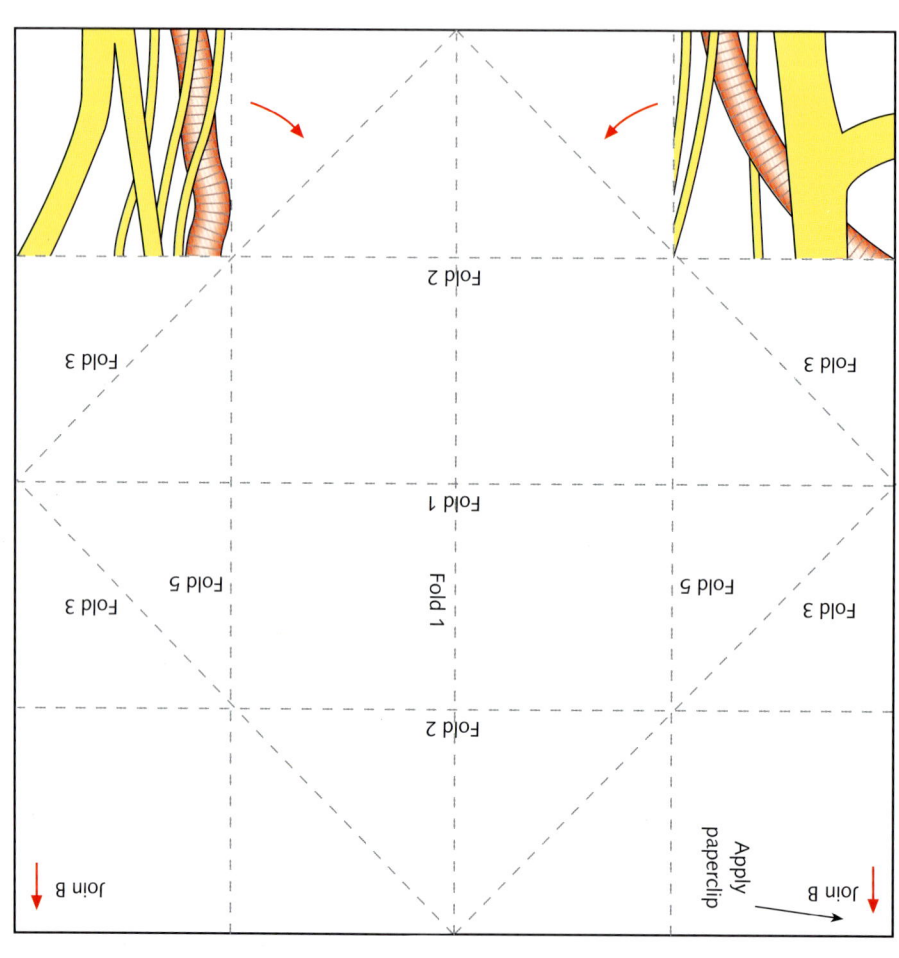

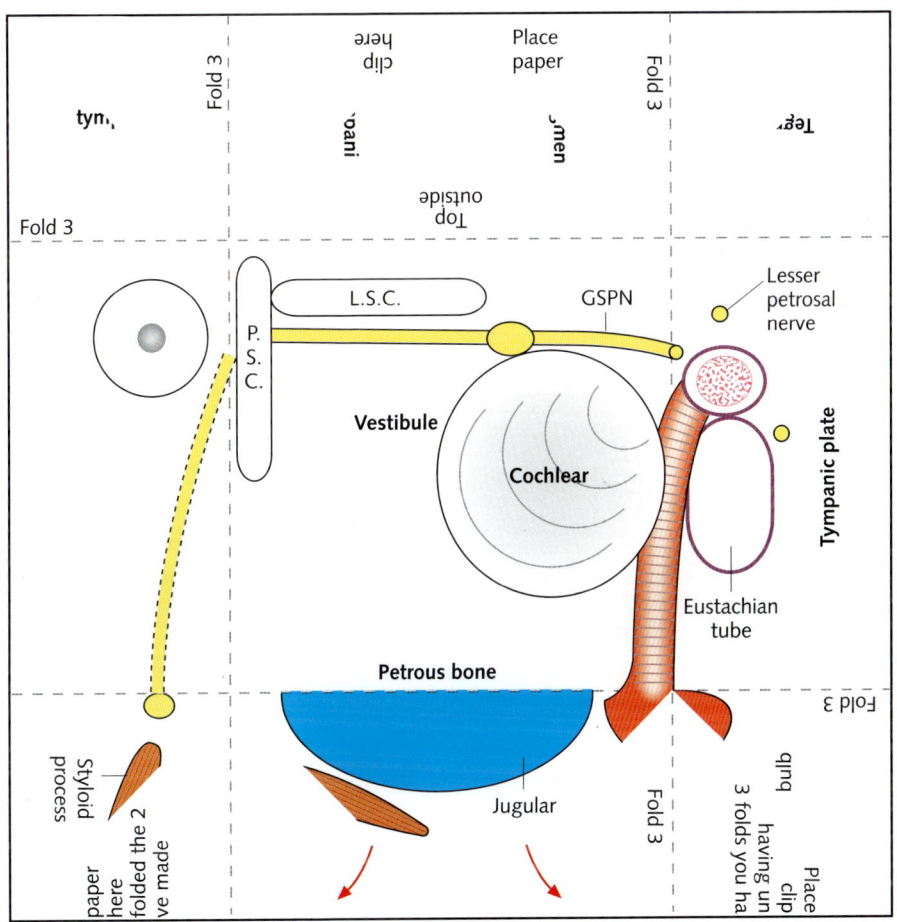

Plate 2 Origami of the middle ear cavity. Cut along outside lines, and fold as instructed.

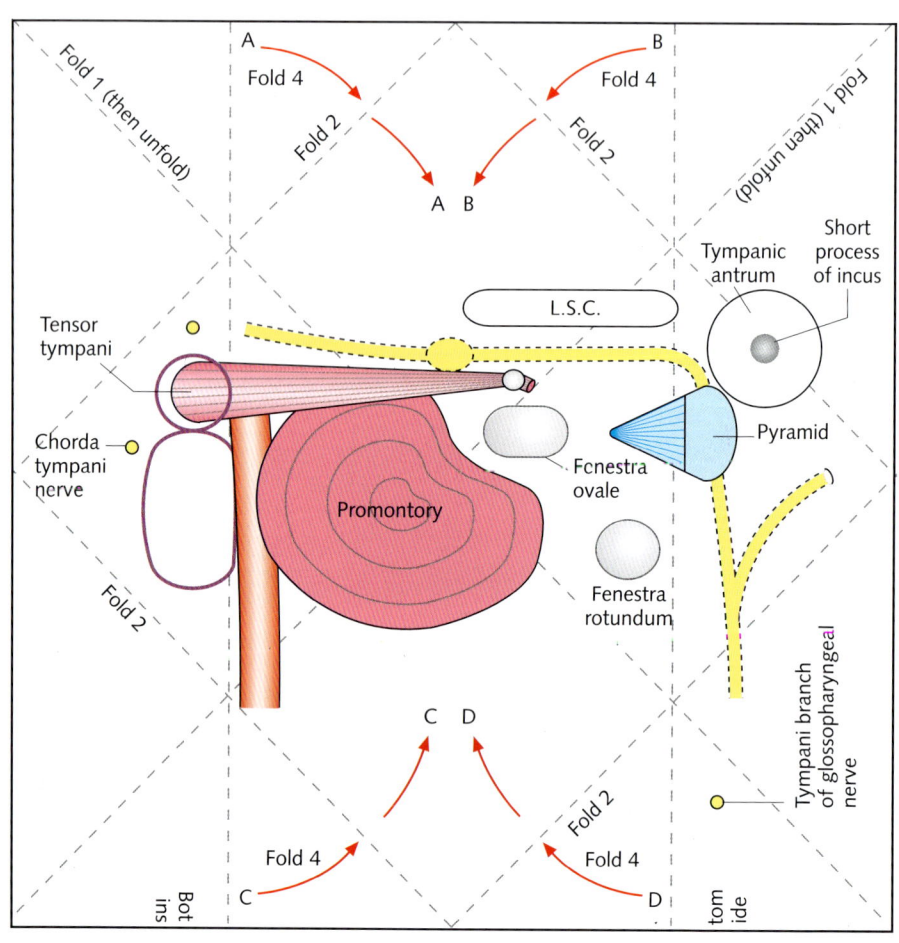

A   B

Fold 4   Fold 4

Fold 1 (then unfold)

Fold 2   Fold 2

Fold 1 (then unfold)

A   B

Tympanic antrum   Short process of incus

L.S.C.

Tensor tympani

Chorda tympani nerve

Pyramid

Promontory

Fenestra ovale

Fenestra rotundum

Fold 2

Tympani branch of glossopharyngeal nerve

C   D

Fold 4   Fold 2   Fold 4

C   D

Bot ins   tom ide

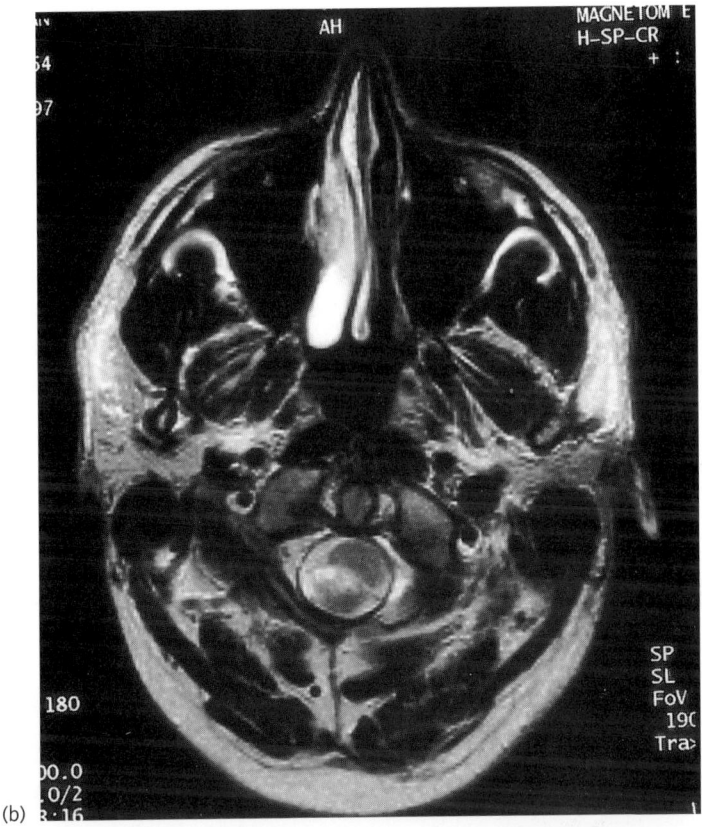

(b)

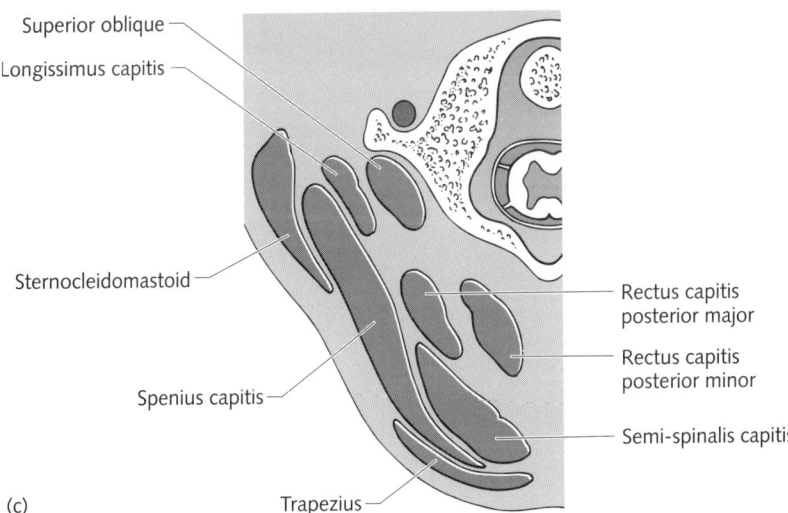

(c)

Fig. 3 (*Continued*) (b) MRI scan to show muscles in cross section. Note the foramen magnum tumour in the spinal canal causing the patient to slightly twist his neck. (c) Diagram of MRI to identify muscles.

parallel line to that formed by the Eustachian tube (and the greater superficial petrosal nerve) and the carotid canal. Hence, tracing the middle meningeal artery back to the foramen spinosum will reveal the greater superficial petrosal nerve which in turn will signify the carotid canal. Occasionally the geniculate ganglion of the facial nerve (from which the greater superficial petrosal nerve arises) may have no bony cover and is vulnerable either to direct trauma or traction trauma via the nerve. Care is required! (See also Figure 15, pp. 22–24.)

I have found it useful to remember, when approaching the cavernous sinus extradurally, that the superior orbital fissure, foramen rotundum, foramen ovale and foramen spinosum create a gentle curve when a line is drawn through these four points.

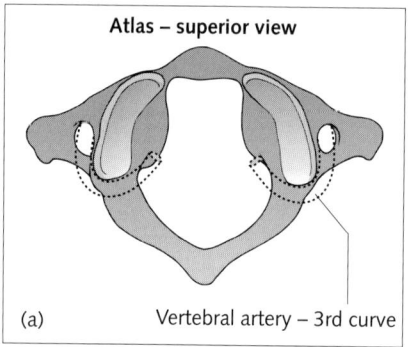

Atlas – superior view

(a)   Vertebral artery – 3rd curve

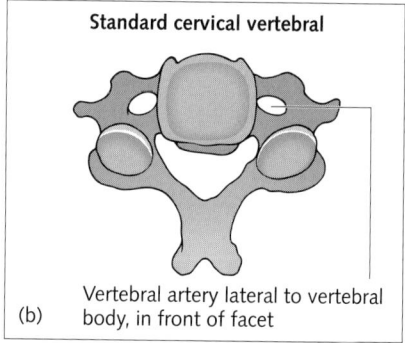

Standard cervical vertebral

(b)   Vertebral artery lateral to vertebral body, in front of facet

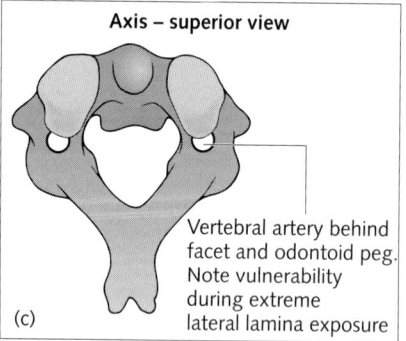

Axis – superior view

(c)   Vertebral artery behind facet and odontoid peg. Note vulnerability during extreme lateral lamina exposure

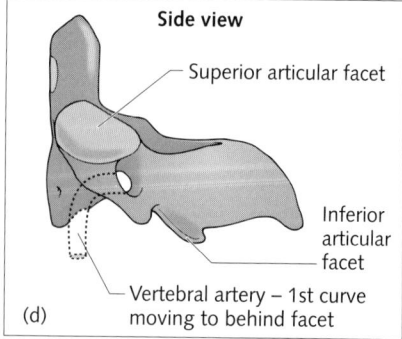

Side view

Superior articular facet

Inferior articular facet

Vertebral artery – 1st curve moving to behind facet

(d)

Fig. 4 (a–d) Diagrams to show the curves of the vertebral artery as it passes from the C3 vertebra (b) to the axis (c and d) and from there to the atlas. The artery is particularly vulnerable as it passes upwards and laterally between C2 and C1 during operations. (*Continued*)

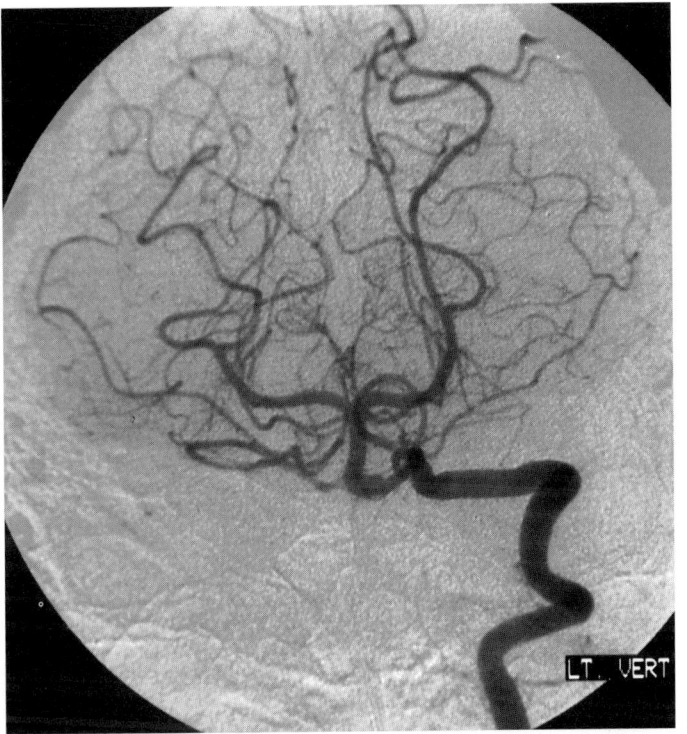

(e)

Fig. 4 (*Continued*) (e) Shows the vertebral artery angiogram in the neck. Work out the three curves yourself!

Cavernous sinus

The cavernous sinus is another important anatomical gold mine. It is actually more like a 'purse' applied to either side of the sella turcica extending from the apex of the petrous bone to the superior orbital fissure. It is tilted so that its lateral extent runs in the line joining the foramen ovale and the foramen rotundum. We at the Radcliffe Infirmary have an 'origami session' to help learn the anatomy of the cavernous sinus, and enclosed in this notebook is an appropriate sheet of paper to allow you to do the same (Plate 1, between pp. 6 and 7). The structures are unmarked to allow you to work out the various nerves. I have found only one nemonic to be useful in the entire field of anatomy and that is for the structures passing through the superior orbital fissure (Figure 5). The tarts are not the edible variety, and it is important to have a reverential pause after the word 'tarts' to signify that the structures have now moved to within the common tendinous origin of the orbital muscles!

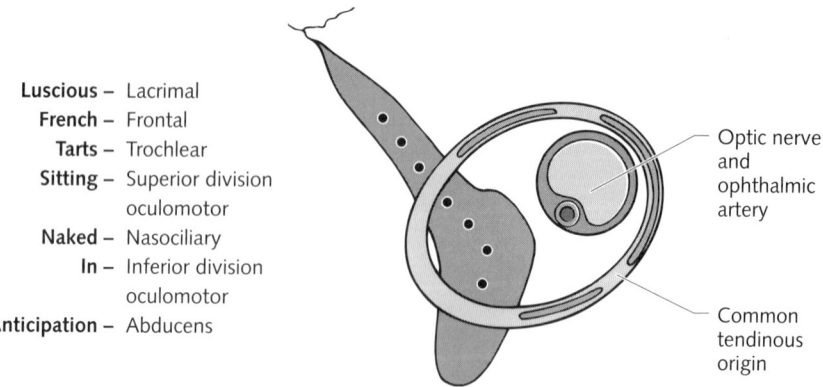

Luscious – Lacrimal
French – Frontal
Tarts – Trochlear
Sitting – Superior division
oculomotor
Naked – Nasociliary
In – Inferior division
oculomotor
Anticipation – Abducens

Optic nerve
and
ophthalmic
artery

Common
tendinous
origin

Fig. 5 Diagram to show the structures passing through the superior orbital fissure.

Middle ear cavity

A game of origami may help with the anatomy of the middle ear (Plate 2, between pp. 6 and 7), which is useful for the neurosurgeon to know even though this is the territory of the otological surgeon. If the trainee knows all these diagrams thoroughly so that they can be produced in his or her mind's eye, then this will be a more than adequate anatomical basis for surgery. Even better would be to make your own diagrams!

Orbital and subtemporal region

Before we leave the skull base it is again useful to have a simple diagram of the orbital and subtemporal region, including the sphenopalatine fossa (Figures 6 and 7). It is essential to know the relationships of the sphenoid wing, but this is usually a familiar area to neurosurgeons. It is the less familiar that I wish to stress.

Grid revision

An excellent exercise is to examine a series of 'bone window' CT scans and identify all the structures on these with those of the grid (Figures 8–12).

Rhomboid

Fukishima has described a 'rhomboid construct', which provides useful

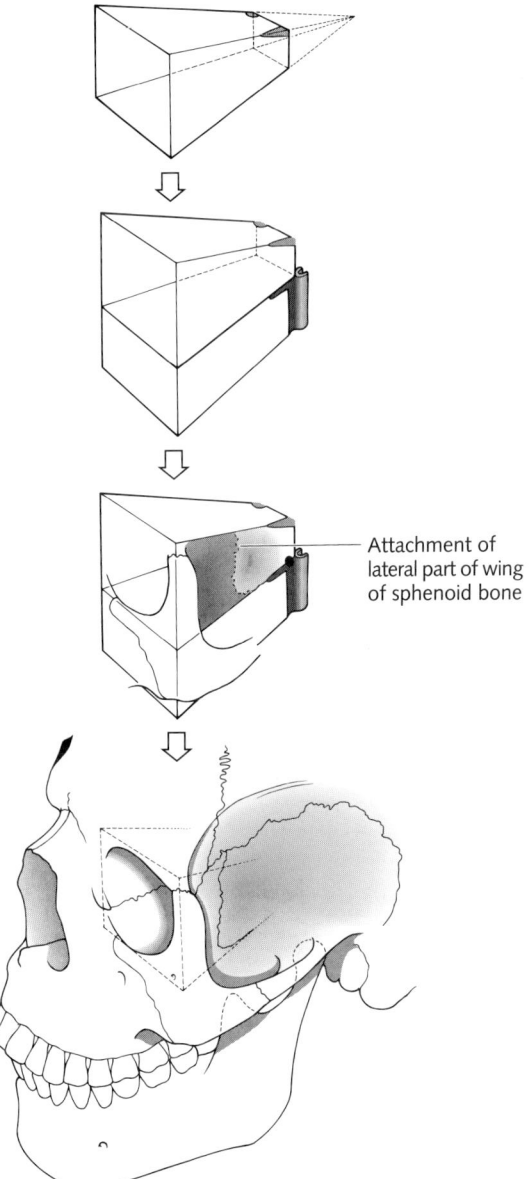

Attachment of
lateral part of wing
of sphenoid bone

Fig. 6 Diagrammatic development of the anterior part of the skull and orbit. The orbit
should be considered as a truncated pyramid. The apex is the superior orbital fissure. The
optic foramen penetrates the superior and medial corner of the truncated apex and the
superior orbital fissure extends between the roof and the lateral wall of the orbit. The
inferior orbital fissure and foramen rotundum is placed between the lateral wall and the
floor of the orbit, while the internal carotid artery grooves the inferior and medial corner
of the truncated apex. From this basic structure the maxilla and the zygomatic bones can
be added, and finally the mandible to produce temporal and subtemporal fossae.

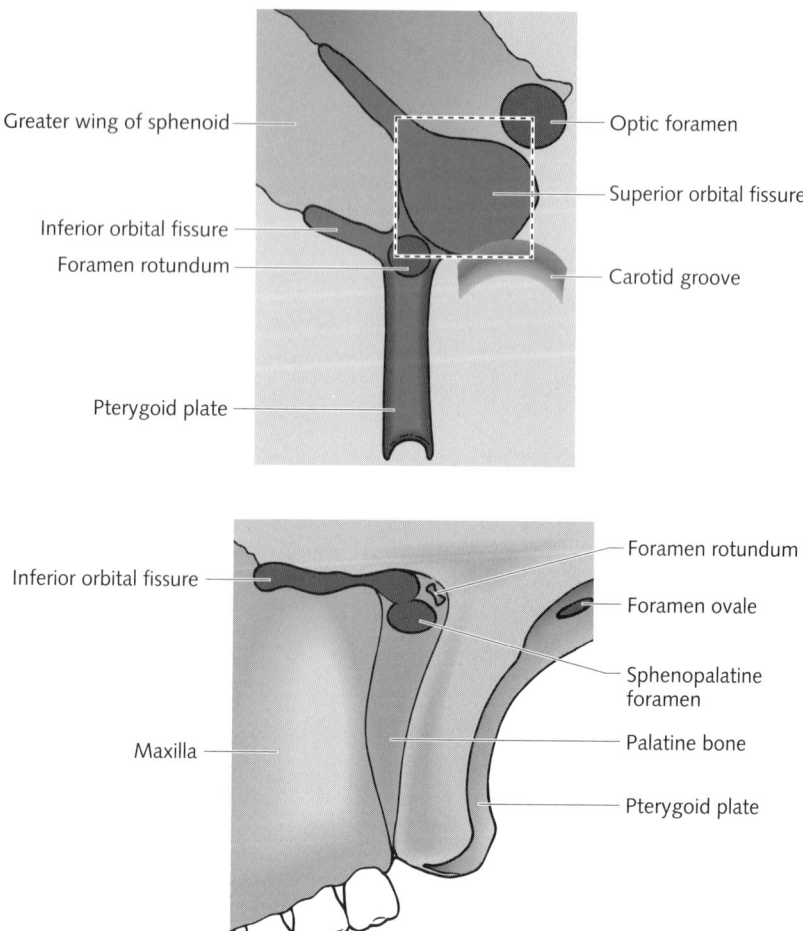

Fig. 7 Diagrams to show the details of the orbital apex and the pterygopalatine fossa. The apex of the orbit is represented by the superior orbital fissure. Each corner of this truncated apex is involved with a hole or a groove (i.e. (clockwise) optic nerve foramen, groove for carotid artery, foramen rotundum, superior orbital fissure).

anatomical knowledge. Figure 13(a) shows this in diagrammatic form (the petrous bone is viewed from above). Compare this with the MRI and CT scans (Figure 13(b–d)).

Surface anatomy

A surgical friend of mine was late for a social event. When asked if the operation had been difficult, he replied, 'the operation was easy but the hole was

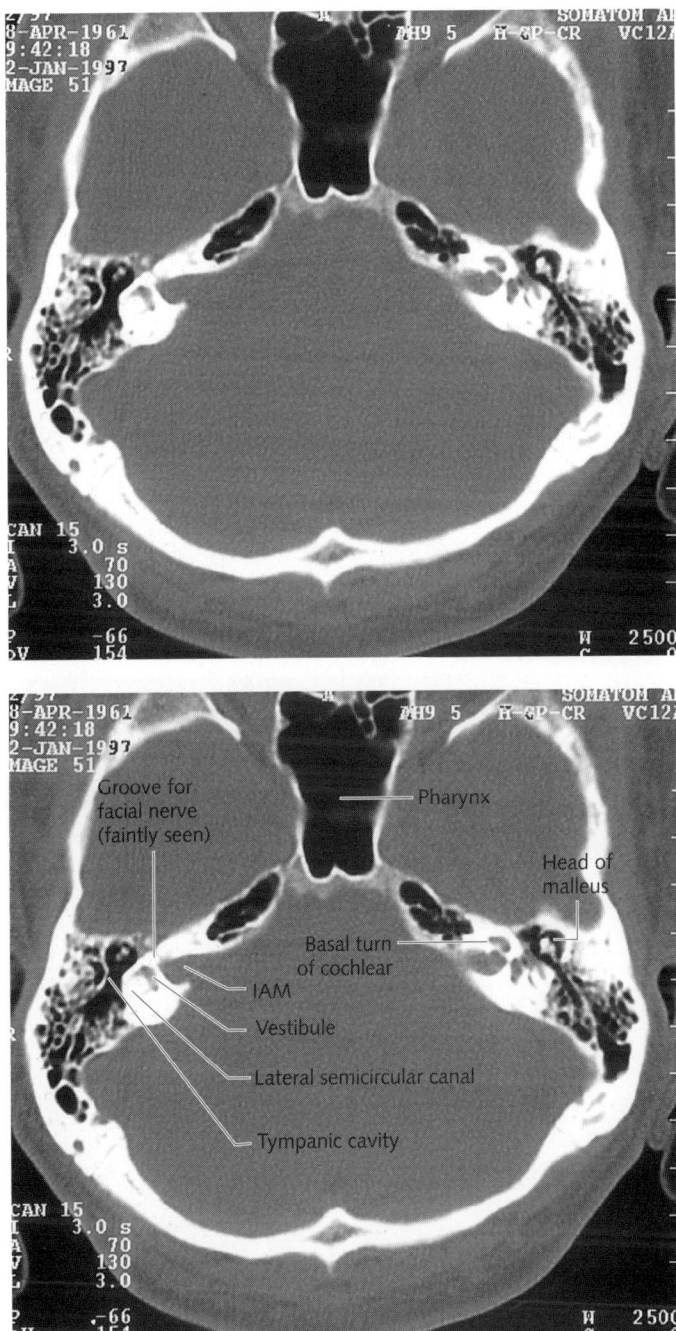

Figs 8–12 Bone window CT scans and maps to revise the skull base grid.

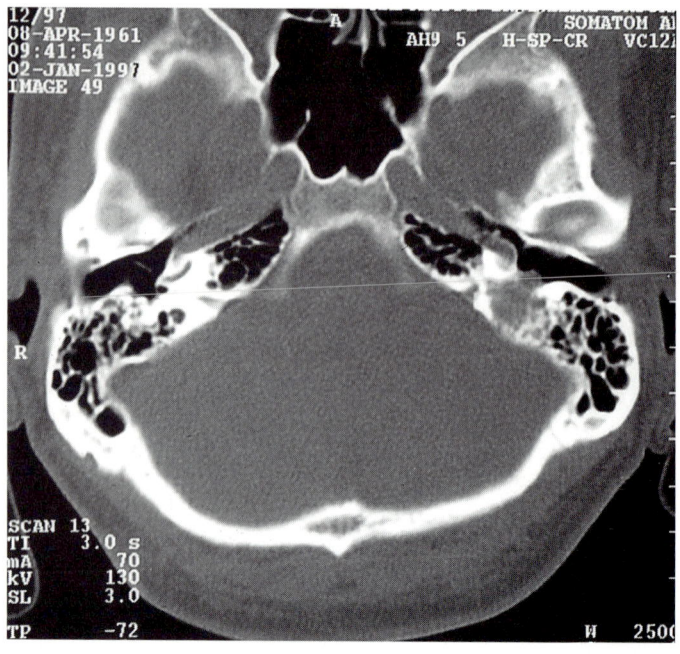

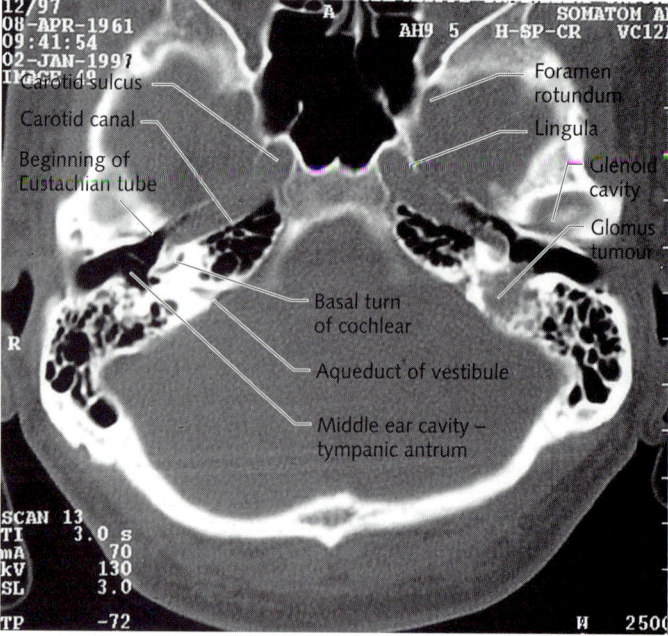

Figs 8–12 (*Continued*)

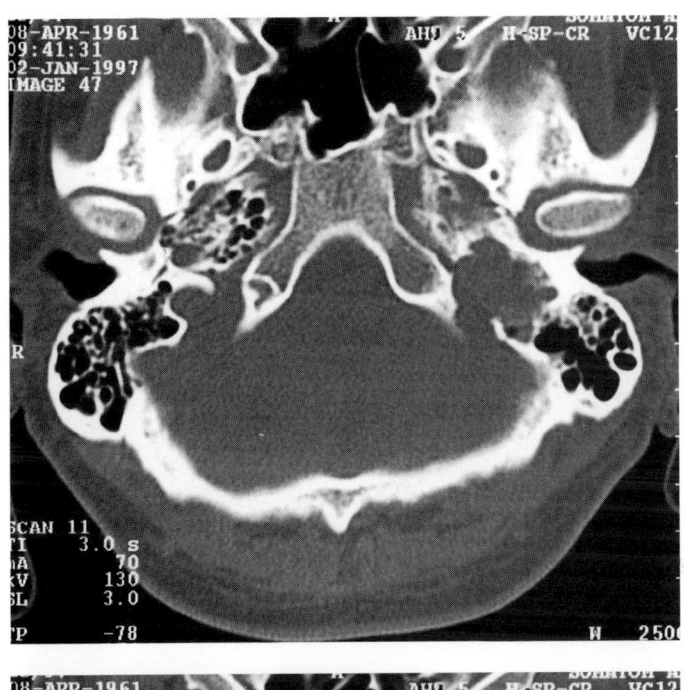

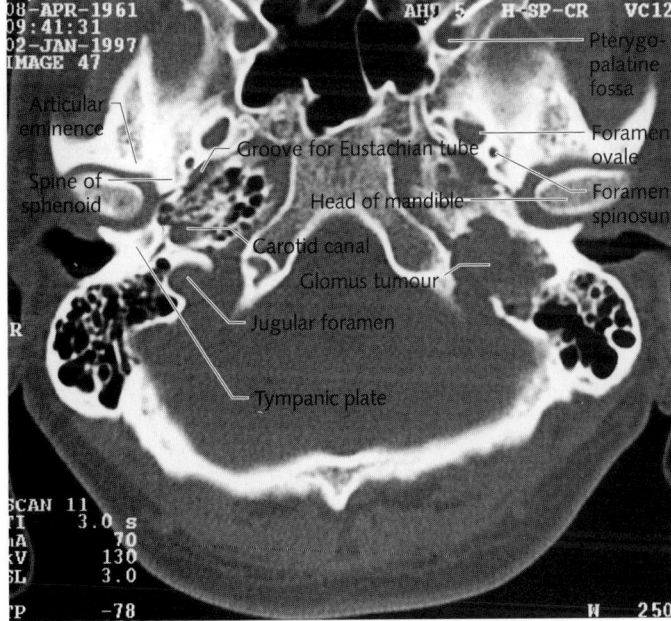

(10)

Figs 8–12 (*Continued*)

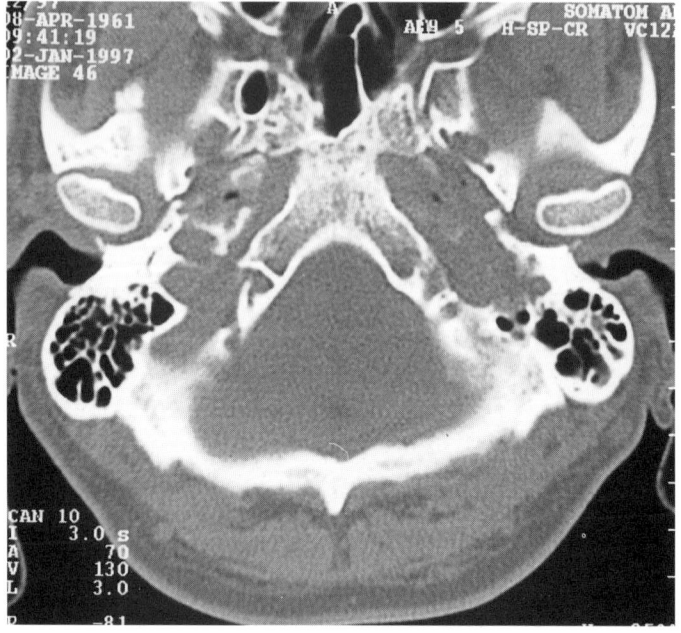

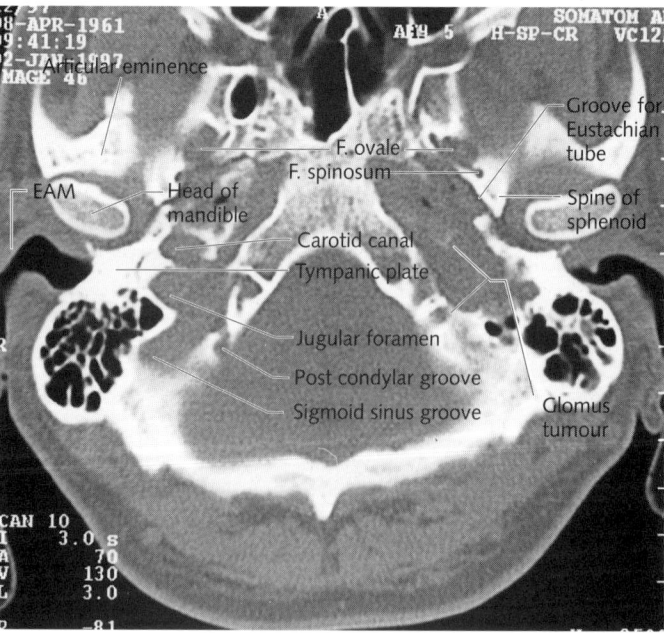

Figs 8–12 (*Continued*)

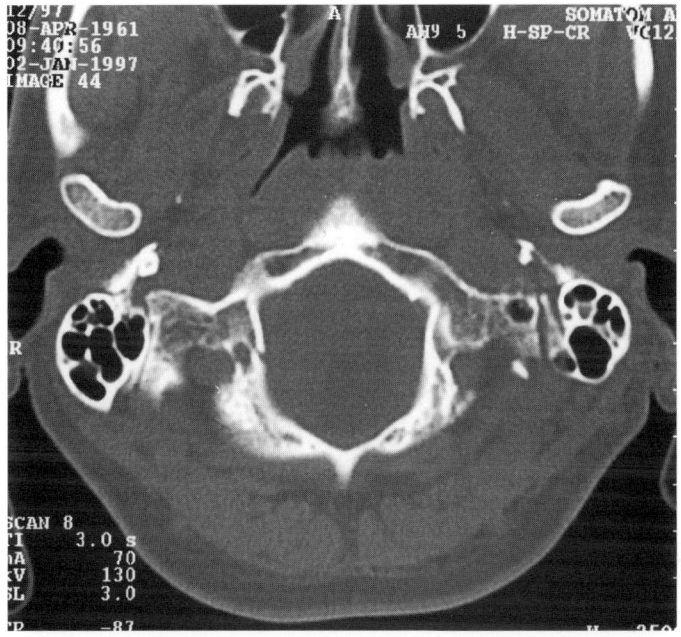

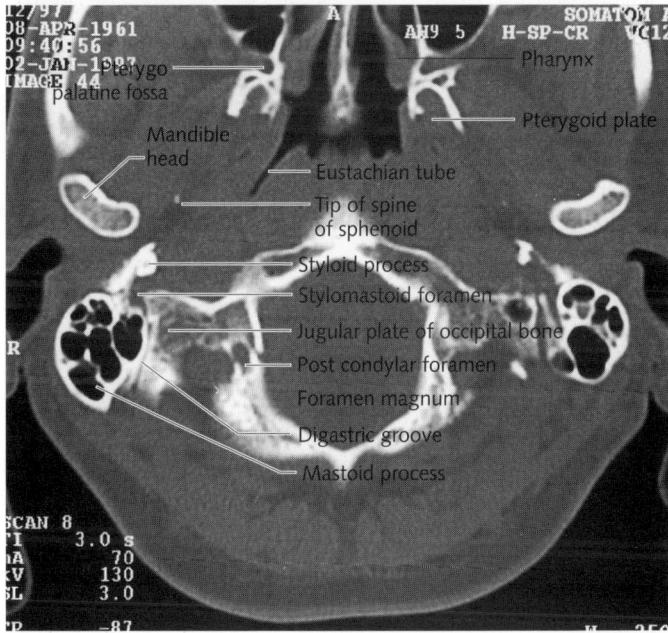

Figs 8–12 (*Continued*)

(12)

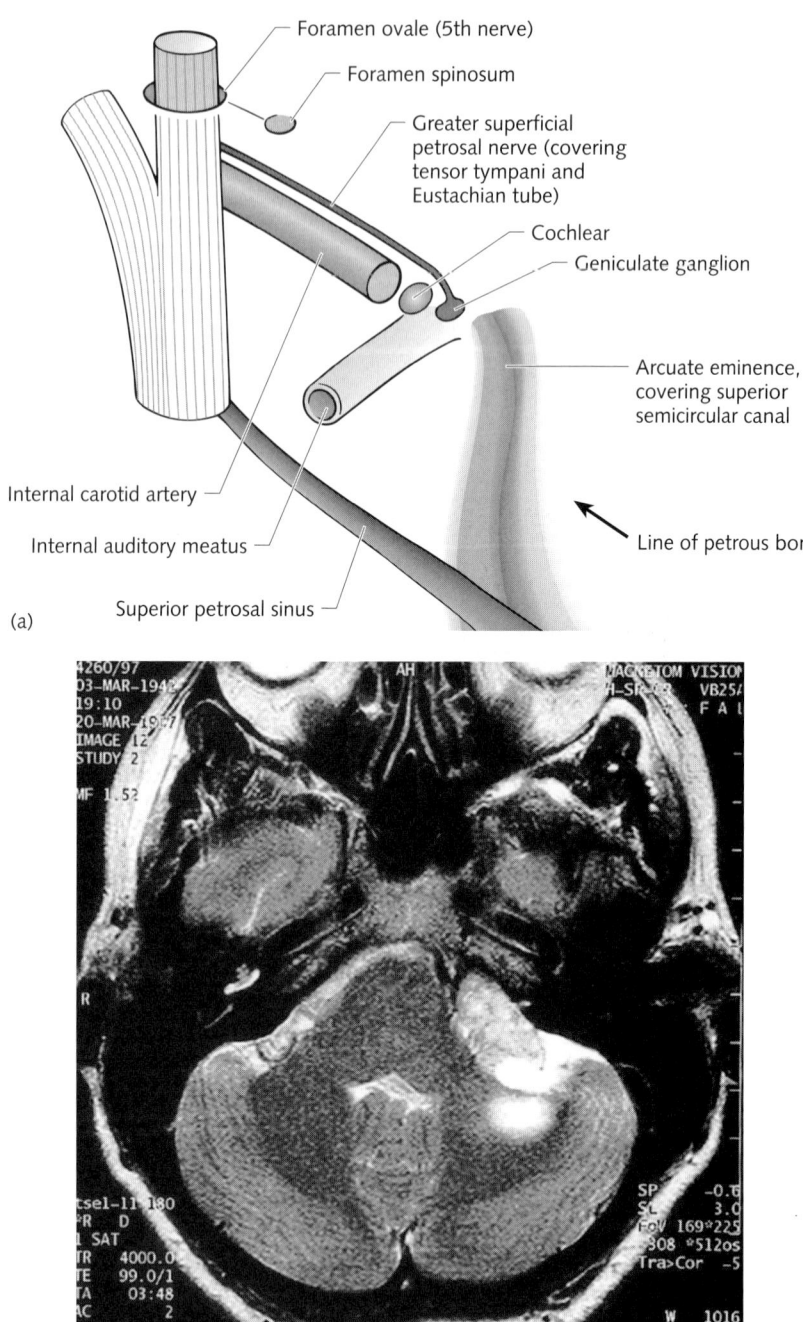

(a)

(b)

Fig. 13 'Useful rhomboid' when drilling off the apex of petrous bone or approaching the IAM through the middle fossa approach. (a) Diagram (after Fukishima). (b) MRI scan to show the (right) carotid canal, cochlea and posterior semicircular canal. (*Continued*)

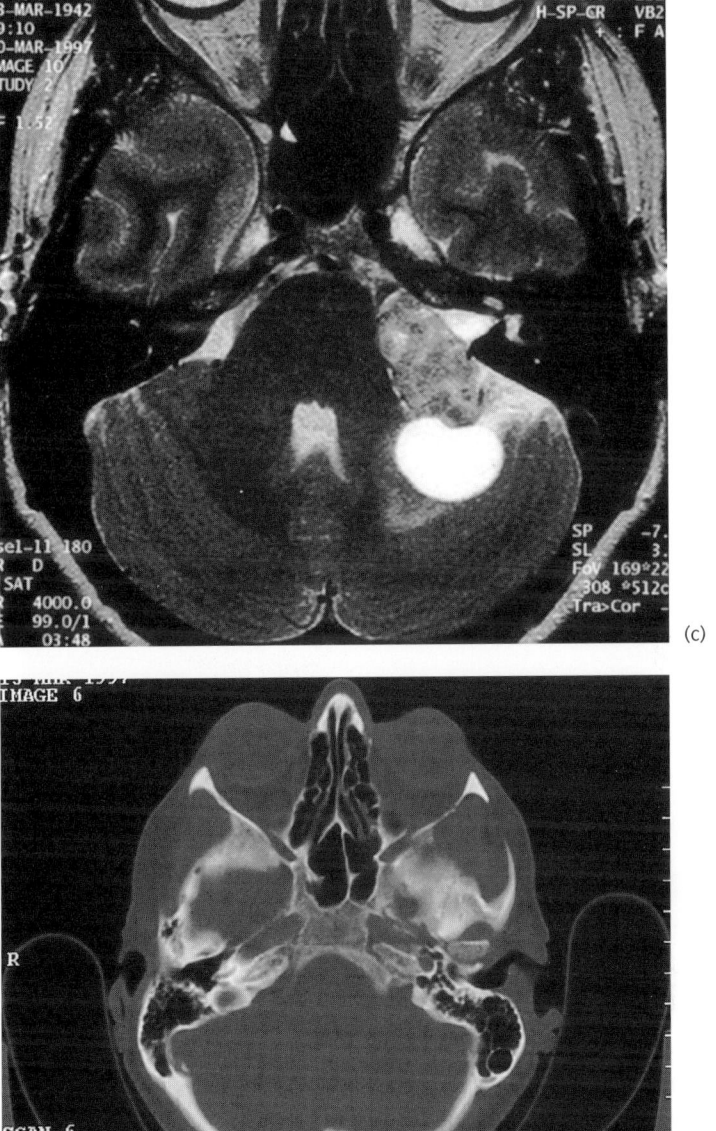

(c)

(d)

Fig. 13 (*Continued*) (c) MRI scan to show the cut ends of the superior semicircular canal (laterally) and the fifth nerve and Meckel's cave (medially). The IAM can be seen inferiorly. (d) CT scan (bone window) to show carotid canal, cochlea, middle ear cavity and Eustachian tube and canal for the endolymphatic duct. This patient had a medially arising, cystic, left acoustic neuroma. The curious dilated IAM without apparent tumour is explained by the cystic extension of the tumour. This proved a most unpleasant tumour to remove. I was unable to spare the facial nerve as it was remarkably stuck to the tumour at the brain stem (due to its medial origin), whereas normally the facial nerve is most adherent just medial to the lip of the IAM (see Figure 52, pp. 154–156).

in the wrong place'. Time taken positioning the patient and carefully working out where the incision should be is time well spent!

Even though stereotaxy and the operating arm system can be of enormous value in localizing lesions, the surgeon still needs to know some surface anatomy in order to carry out common operative procedures. The most useful is the coronal suture which is 3–4 cm in front of the central sulcus. If the surgeon stays anterior to the coronal suture, he or she will not be endangering the motor cortex. I find the best way of finding the coronal suture is to place the tip of my index finger on the eyebrow, and my knuckles indicate the coronal suture at the midline. This distance is 11 cm (Figure 14). The motor cortex or strip is best defined by marking the midpoint between the root of the nose and the external occipital protuberance. A point 1 cm behind this midpoint marks the central sulcus at the midline, and a line three-quarters of a right angle from this (i.e. 67.5°) indicates the line of the central sulcus passing forwards and laterally.

The Sylvian fissure starts at the pterion (in a line 45° from the frontozygomatic suture). The fissure is approximately one-third of the distance from the floor of the middle fossa to the sagittal suture. It is important for the surgeon to know that the floor of the middle fossa is indicated by the zygomatic arch and the floor of the anterior cranial fossa is at the frontozygomatic suture.

The pinna of the ear is a useful marker when using the MRI scan. It is well seen on the scan, and temporal tumours can be easily related to the tip of the pinna. The brain stem is roughly between two lines joining in the front and the back of the right and left pinnas. Those who needle the trigeminal nerve will know that the foramen ovale lies 2.5 cm in front of the external auditory meatus (as does the posterior clinoid process and hence the anterior aspect of the third ventricle).

Detecting the central sulcus on scans

It is important to know where the central sulcus (and hence motor cortex and speech areas) is on the MRI scans. Figure 15(a) illustrates on a lateral view the relevant sulci and gyri, whereas Figure 15(b) and (c) show the 'bracket sign' for the central sulcus at the vertex. Both CT and MRI scans are used to illustrate this sign and the reference for this important information is given at the end of the book (Naidich & Brightbill, 1996). I urge you to consult the original article.

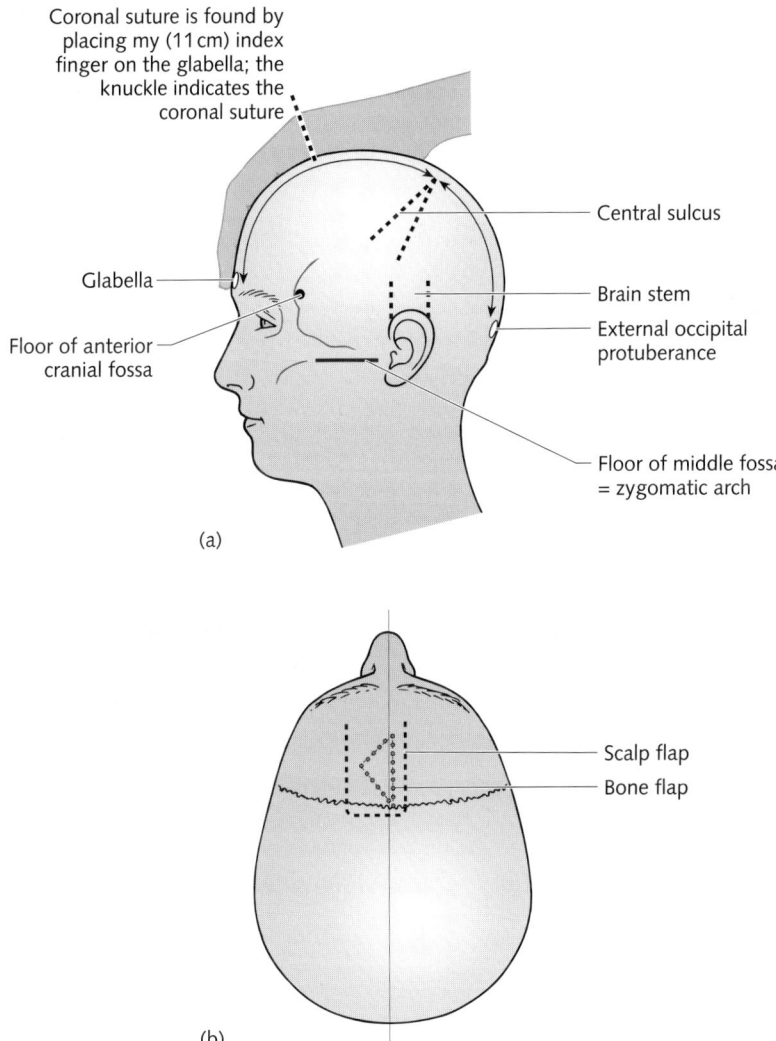

Coronal suture is found by placing my (11 cm) index finger on the glabella; the knuckle indicates the coronal suture

Central sulcus

Glabella

Brain stem

Floor of anterior cranial fossa

External occipital protuberance

Floor of middle fossa = zygomatic arch

(a)

Scalp flap
Bone flap

(b)

Fig. 14 (a) Useful surface markings of the head. Use the MRI scan. One can identify the coronal suture on a sagittal MRI scan. One can see the pinna of the ear on the coronal and axial scans. Use the coronal suture and the pinna to guide you. I often use a ruler to make measurements on the MRI scan and then, using the centimetre scale on the scan, transfer these measurements to the head of the patient. This can be a remarkably accurate way of defining where a lesion is. Try it! The central sulcus at the midline is three-quarters of a right angle from 1 cm behind the midpoint between the glabella and the external occipital protuberance. (b) Diagram to show a parasagittal scalp incision for a transcallosal approach to the third ventricle. It is important to place the medial incision 1 cm across the midline so that the dural opening can be flush with the sagittal sinus so avoiding any brain retraction. The triangular bone flap is indicated.

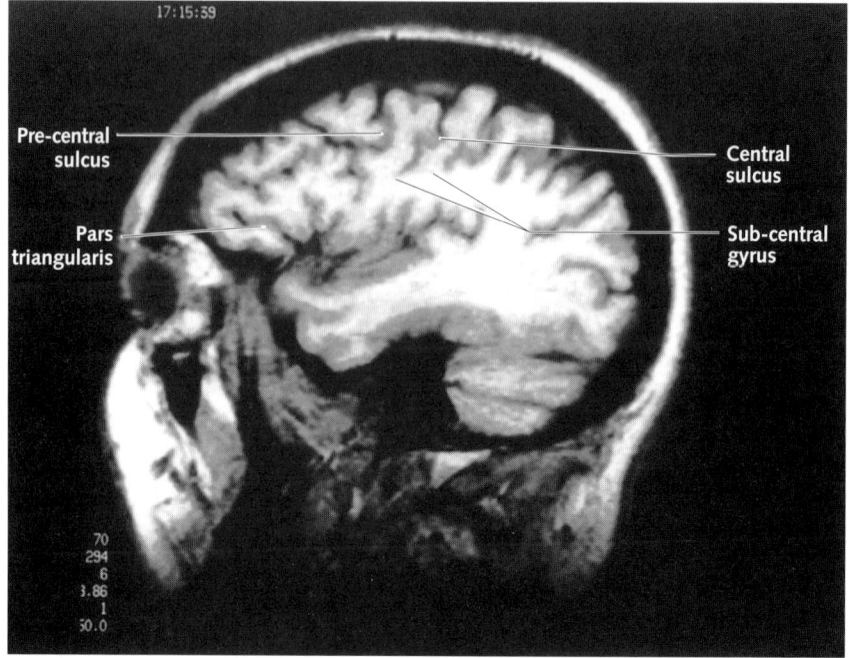

Fig. 15 (a) A lateral MRI scan. First look for the pars triangularis in the inferior frontal gyrus. Then find the (oblique) pre-central sulcus (often in two parts) and then the central sulcus, which never meets the Sylvian fissure but is separated by a 'sub-central' gyrus. The post-central sulcus is behind and parallel to the central sulcus and these define the motor and sensory cortex. The two speech areas are in practice quite variable but are in the dominant inferior frontal gyrus and in the area where the Sylvian fissure terminates in the inferior parietal lobule (angular gyrus). I refer you to George Ojemann's article in Further reading. (*Continued*)

Spinal anatomy

Cervical spine

The vertebral artery

The 'three curves' of the vertebral artery are most important and this information is perhaps insufficiently emphasized. Some authors make it four curves but I will settle for three. The artery is well protected to the inferior

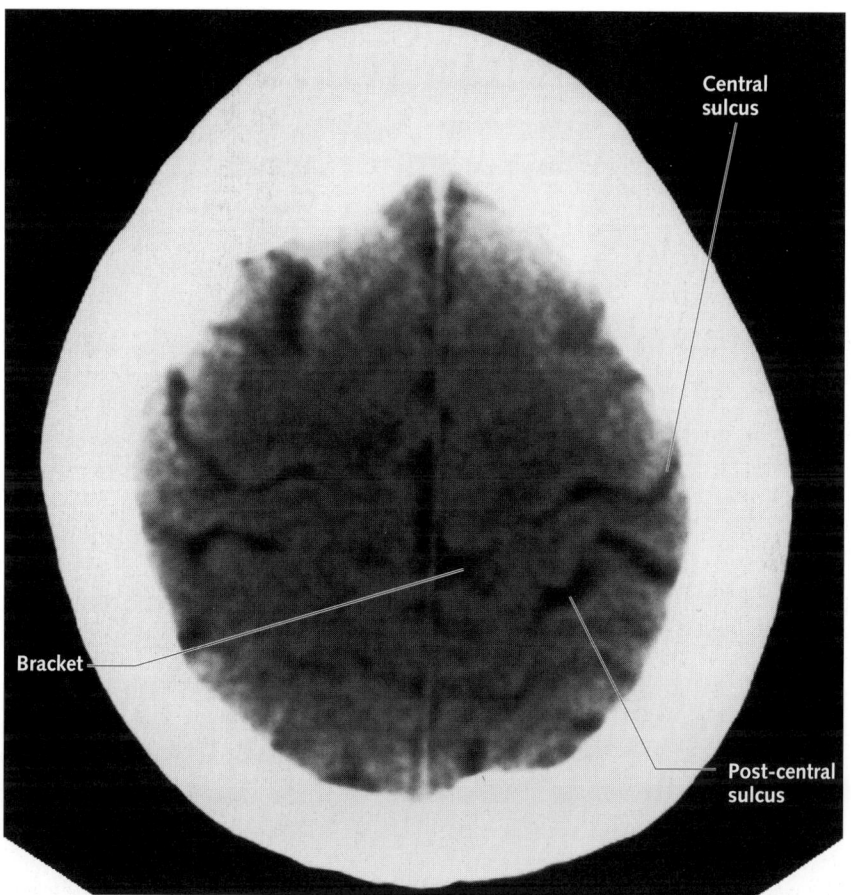

(b)

Fig. 15 (*Continued*) (b,c) The 'bracket sign'. Look for the (widest) biparietal diameter of the skull. Then find the widest midline sulcus, usually placed at the widest diameter of the skull. The post-central sulcus bifurcates as it approaches the 'bracket'. The central sulcus is just in front. Because of the different scanning angles of CT and MRI, often the bracket sign is more centrally placed on the CT scan and hence easier to see. (*Continued* on p. 24)

aspect of the C2 vertebra, but is especially vulnerable passing from C2 to the transverse process of C1. The first curve occurs when the vertebral artery passes from its usual position lateral to the vertebral body backwards, upwards and laterally to emerge posterior to the 'sloping shoulders'— superior articular facet of C2. The second curve occurs upwards, laterally

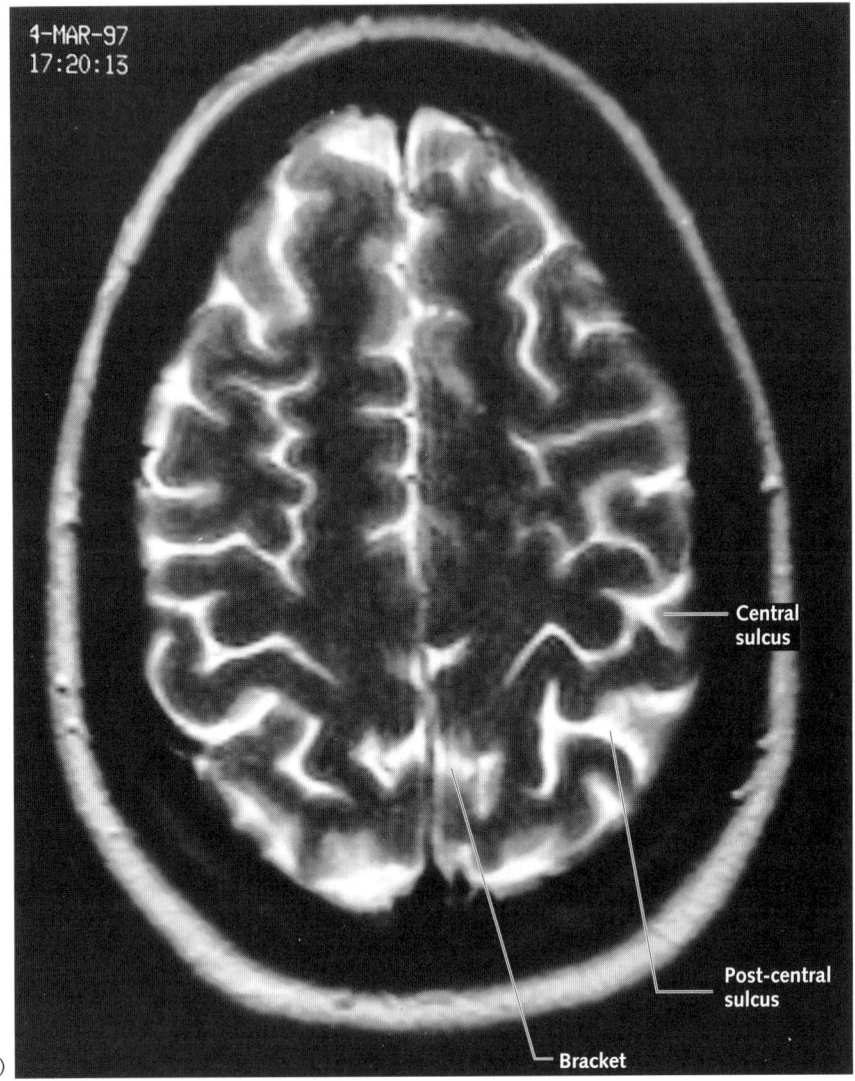

4-MAR-97
17:20:13

Central sulcus

Post-central sulcus

Bracket

(c)

Fig. 15 (*Continued*)

and forwards to enter the foramen of C1 transverse process. This curve is related to the C2 nerve which is a useful landmark and the artery is covered here by the splenius cervicalis muscle. Note the vertebral artery may well be damaged by the far lateral exposure of the lamina of C2, during a cervical laminectomy, unlike more caudally in the cervical spine. The third vertebral artery curve is almost a complete semicircle around the superior articular facet of C1. Look at an MRI scan to appreciate how near a semicircle this is. When carrying out a midline exposure of the posterior fossa, the vertebral artery is best exposed (having exposed the tubercle of the posterior arch of C1) by 'pushing' a mastoid strip along the upper border of the arch. Often a small 'dead space' is revealed around the vertebral artery before finding the venous plexus which intimately surrounds the vertebral artery.

Look at a C2 vertebra; the artery enters it (from C3) pointing vertically but leaves it almost laterally. This vertebral artery curve is very acute being roughly 70° in both the transverse and antero-posterior planes, as it emerges from the C2 foramen to pass up to C1 (see Figure 4).

The third, final curve of the vertebral artery is around the superior articular facet of C1. Look at this bone if you have one. This facet is centred at the midpoint between the tip of the transverse process of C1 and the tubercle marking the midline point of the posterior arch of C1. In other words, this semicircular curve of the vertebral artery is in the middle of each half of C1 when viewed from behind. Intimate knowledge of this artery is needed for the lateral approaches for foramen magnum tumours (antero-lateral and postero-lateral: see George & Lot (1995) in the Further reading section).

By the way, do you know the six muscles arising from the transverse process of C1? Figure 3 will help with four; the other two are the levator scapulae and the scalenus medius. These two muscles are continuous with the splenius capitis and all three form the floor of the posterior triangle of the neck. 'Splenius' is my favourite muscle name; it means a bandage, and the splenius capitis is a broad, flat muscle applied obliquely to the back of the neck, just like a bandage. Look it up in an anatomical textbook.

We do not fully understand the functional changes in the vertebral arteries with neck posture. A colleague of mine once did a Dandy McKenzie operation on a woman with persistent (not spasmodic) torticollis. A few hours post-operation she developed pontine ischaemia (not medullary). I surmised that the persistent torticollis had allowed one vertebral artery to stretch and the other to shorten. When the head was straightened after many years of being twisted, the stretched artery kinked and the shortened one stretched, thus causing brain-stem ischaemia. By the way, if you do this operation warn the patient that there may be post-operative dysphagia: you need to extend the head to swallow (try it!) and this operation if done bilaterally and extensively may make this difficult. We do not know the cause of this condition and this operation merely weakens the neck muscles. Not a good answer, but if the patient gets fed up with botulinum injections then it is probably the next safest procedure to try.

Thoracic spine

The relationship of the ribs to the vertebral arteries and intercostal nerves can easily cause confusion and needs to be remembered when carrying out a trans-thoracic approach or an antero-lateral costotransversectomy approach to a thoracic disc prolapse. I have given up the latter approach doing either a trans-thoracic approach for a central thoracic disc prolapse or a postero-lateral trans-pedicular approach for a more unilateral thoracic disc prolapse. Figure 16 clarifies the relationships between the vertebral bodies, the ribs and the intercostal nerves, which I find particularly confusing.

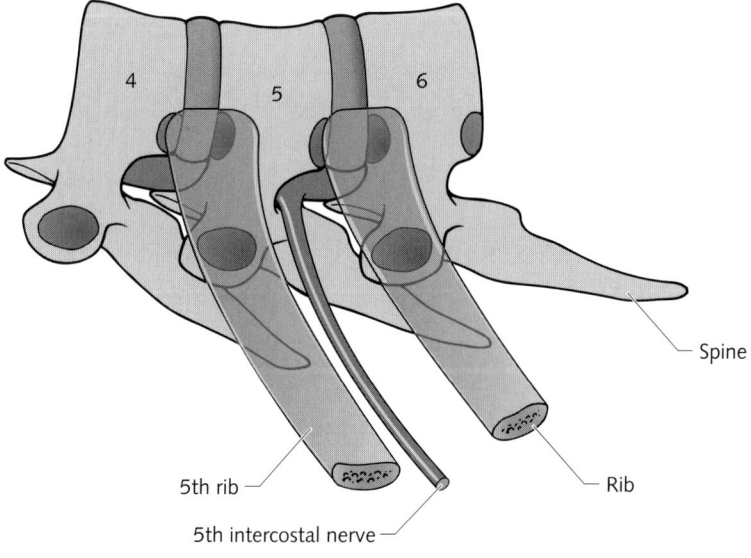

NB	5th rib straddles T4 and T5 vertebral bodies (and disc)
	5th intercostal nerve (and nerve root) emerges between T5 and T6 and runs below T5 rib

Fig. 16 Thoracic spine. Diagram to show the relationship between the vertebral bodies, the ribs and intercostal nerves. This information is essential when carrying out a trans-thoracic or costotransversectomy approach to a thoracic disc protrusion. I find the numbering of the different structures very confusing and I always remind myself of these relationships before tackling a thoracic disc prolapse. I have stopped using the costotransversectomy approach.

Lumbar spine

The best way to remember which nerve is related to which vertebra is to realize that the nerve root hugs the pedicle of the vertebra of the same number. Hence the L5 nerve root hugs the pedicle of L5 and so on. It is often useful if one has to find a nerve root to first find the pedicle (Figure 17). How do you find the pedicle? In the lumbar region a line drawn through the cranial border of the spinous process passes through the superior articular facet, the pedicle and the transverse process. This is also useful information if you wish to carry out a fusion (see Figure 18).

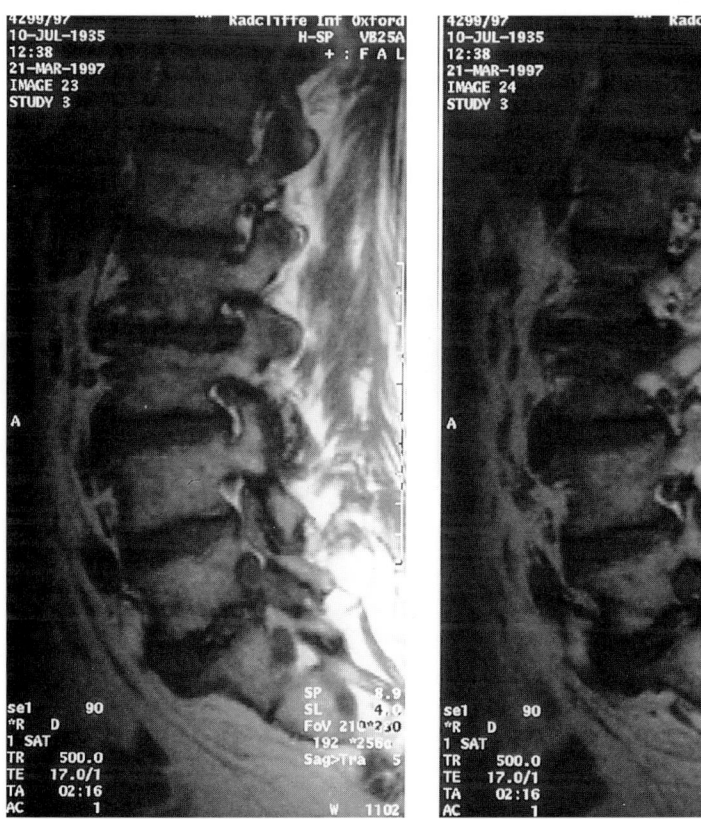

Fig. 17 MRI scan to show compression of the L5 nerve as it passes beneath the pedicle of L5 at the L5 S1 level. Notice the normal pear-shaped foramina with the nerve (adjacent to the pedicle) surrounded by fat (white). The small black dots in the intervertebral foramina are veins. Too often people concentrate on the lumbar discs and fail to study the lateral cuts, which, especially on a T1-weighted sequence (fat is white) shows the foraminal anatomy beautifully.

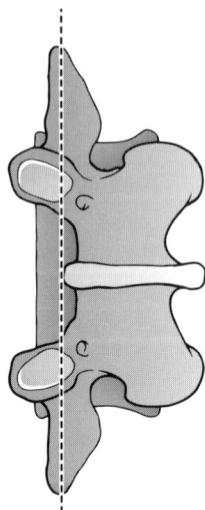

Line drawn along the **upper** (cranial) border of spinous
process runs through the **pedicle**, transverse process
and superior articular facet (lower margin)

Fig. 18 The lumbar spine from above: this diagram emphasizes the importance of the line drawn through the upper (cranial) margin of the spinous process. This line traverses the pedicles, the transverse processes and the lower margin of the superior articular facet. It is important to know where to find the pedicle because this will lead you to the nerve of the same number as the vertebra, i.e. the L5 nerve root curves around the pedicle of the L5 vertebra hugging the pedicle as it emerges through the intervertebral foramen.

chapter three

Tips on taking a history and examining patients

The history

The history tells you the pathology, the examination tells you where the pathology is. If you are stumped by a patient, go back and take the history again. All these statements are true, but there is a real art in taking a history and this art takes time to learn. Like a lawyer, you must obtain the facts (as opposed to your own or the patient's speculation) without asking 'leading questions'. In other words, phrase your questions carefully so they do not suggest an answer to the patient. The only difference between the doctor and the lawyer on this occasion is that the doctor must put the patient at ease and empathize with him or her prior to asking questions. It does not pay, however, to let the patient talk in an uncontrolled manner and it is often advisable to ask questions that have a yes or no answer. For example, instead of asking a patient to describe his or her bladder function, one could ask 'do you get a normal feeling of a full bladder or not?'. In fact, when asking a patient with suspected cauda equina compression I ask three questions. The first is 'do you have a normal feeling of a full bladder?', the second is 'can you feel the urine passing down the urethra?'; if the answer is no, then one asks how the patient knows when he or she has finished passing urine and the answer must be 'when the noise of the urine flowing into the receptacle ceases'. The final question relates to the anal canal mucosal sensitivity and is 'can you differentiate if you are going to pass flatus or faeces?'. All these questions require a yes or no answer and avoid the patient regaling you with intricate details of how little or how much pushing etc. is required, which is of little help in elucidating neurological function.

Sensory symptoms

An experienced clinician uses the history to focus his or her examination.

29

Numbness on its own is an unreliable symptom, often meaning different things to patients and doctors. Pins and needles on the other hand, with or without numbness, is a very reliable symptom, indicating a disorder of the nervous system from the sensory cortex to the peripheral nerve. If the lesion is in the spinal cord, the pins and needles indicate a posterior column abnormality and is often associated with a tightness or gripping ('like a blood-pressure cuff') around the chest, abdomen or legs depending on the level of the lesion. Spino-thalamic tract involvement produces no pins and needles whatsoever; these patients notice a lack of appreciation of pain and temperature and complain of painless injuries. I had one patient who painlessly nailed his forearm to the workbench. An absence of pins and needles may make a posterior column disorder unlikely but one can only exclude a spino-thalamic tract disorder by testing with a pin.

Epilepsy

When recording the history of an epileptic attack or similar disorders, it is best to record what the patient experiences and what an observer saw. Of course it is essential to obtain a history from the relatives when there is a possibility of personality or memory change and similar disorders of 'higher intellectual functioning'.

Pain

When investigating pain obtain as precise a description as possible of the site of the pain as well as the factors increasing or decreasing it, and whether or not there are periods without pain. Always be aware of any pain that wakes a patient at night; it is usually a severe pain. We know the headache of raised intracranial pressure is worse at night or on waking (which may be earlier than usual), but did you know that sciatica waking the patient at night and furthermore forcing the patient out of bed to pace up and down and eventually spend the night sitting in a chair, is typical of cauda equina compression due to a neurofibroma or ependymoma? (Figure 19(a)). Root pain arising higher in the spinal canal, due to a meningioma or neurofibroma, may also wake the patient up at night and force him or her to get out of bed to walk around.

Any interscapular pain, especially waking the patient at night, should be considered to be due to a metastatic deposit until proved otherwise, especially if the patient is known to have a primary lesion elsewhere. I am continually distressed by the number of paraplegic patients that are admitted

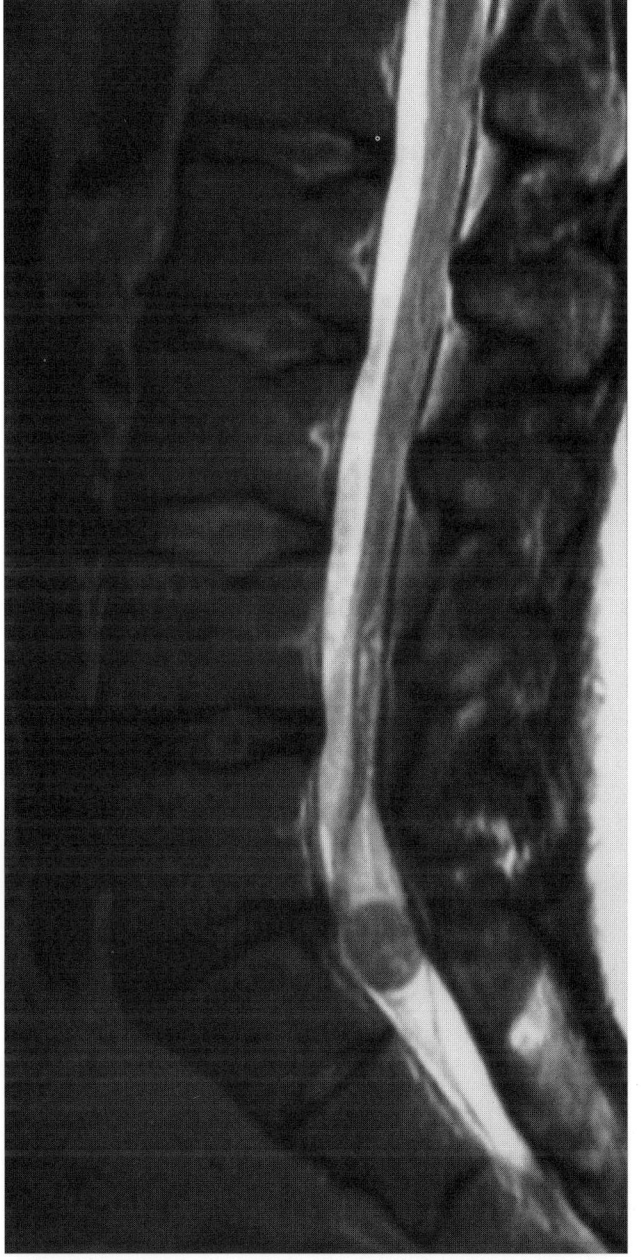

(a)

Fig. 19 Two causes of nocturnal pain. (a) MRI scan of an ependymoma (extradural) in a medical student woken up by severe back pain and bilateral sciatica. He was virtually pain free by day. I removed most but not all of this tumour, as I did not wish to damage bladder, bowel and sexual function. These tumours are radiosensitive and when the nerves are very stuck it is better to resist the temptation to totally remove the tumour. This illustrates well the surgeon's dilemma; discretion is sometimes the better part of valour and knowing when to stop the operation demands judgement and self discipline. (*Continued*)

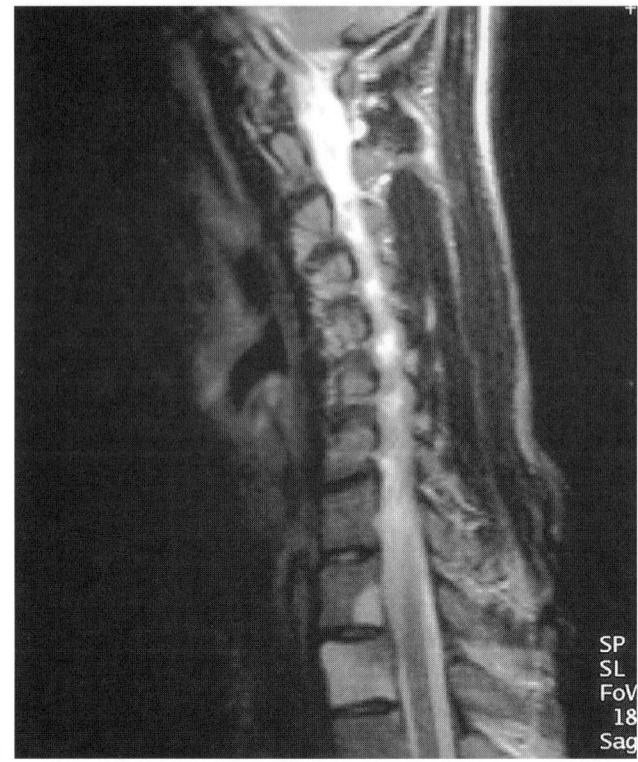

(b)

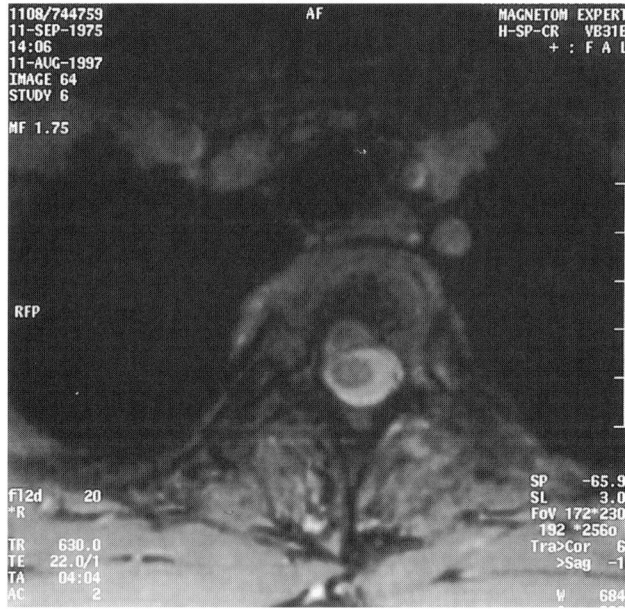

(c)

Fig. 19 (*Continued*) (b–d) Osteoblastoma of T3 vertebral body. (b) MRI scan shows oedema of T3 vertebral body and the adjacent body of T2. Note the actual tumour is placed posterior and superiorly at T3. (c,d) Axial cuts (MRI and CT) to show the osteoblastoma. See text. (*Continued*)

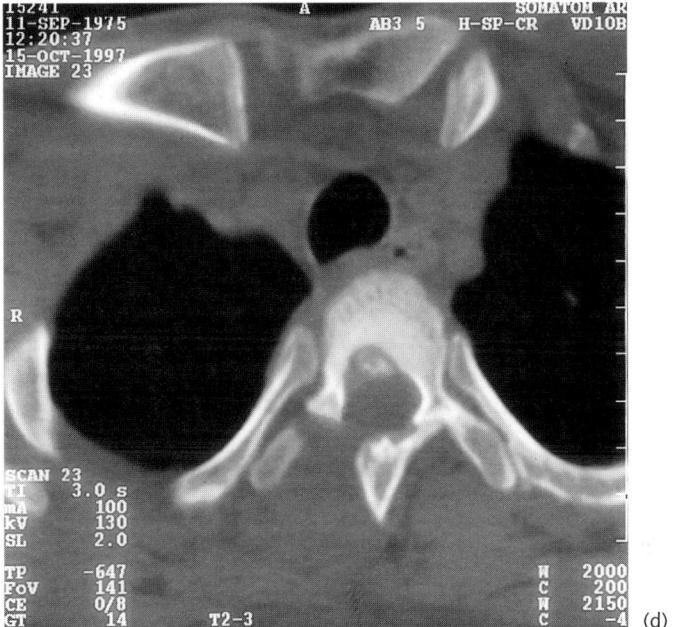

Fig. 19 (*Continued*)

with a long history of interscapular pain which has not been diagnosed; yet how much better it would be for the patient to have the diagnosis made at the 'pain stage', and receive irradiation then and so avoid spinal cord compression. It is said that night pain is typical of an osteoid osteoma of the spine, which responds dramatically to aspirin. I have had one such patient in 30 years, so this condition must be as rare as hens' teeth or I keep missing them! Osteoid osteomas look rather like a polo sweet on the scan, so one is not likely to miss this pathology these days. Perhaps they are just very rare!

Osteoblastomas are near relatives of osteoid osteomas. They cause night pain which is often relieved by aspirin but characteristically cause a lot of surrounding oedema. Figure 19(b–d) shows such a lesion in a Cambridge undergraduate. Two unsuccessful biopsies were attempted elsewhere and successful excision achieved (by a postero-lateral approach removing the pedicle, transverse process and head and neck of the rib) once it was realized the tumour was in fact small and the more obvious lesion was oedema.

Examining the patient

Testing strength

Weakness of dorsiflexion of the foot is the world's most commonly missed physical sign! It is extraordinary that probably 90% of neurologists and neurosurgeons (not to mention orthopaedic surgeons) do not know how to examine for weakness of dorsiflexion of the foot. This is commonly affected with lumbar disc prolapse or lateral recess stenosis, yet this diagnostically important weakness is missed. Why? The reason is that doctors are taught to test for this weakness by asking the patient to 'bend the foot back and keep it there', the doctor subsequently attempting to plantar flex the foot and over-come the patient's attempts to dorsiflex the foot. This method disguises con-siderable weakness because the patient can 'lock' the foot in this position. Much more reliable is to start with the foot plantar flexed and resist the patient's efforts to dorsiflex. In other words 'go with the movement' (Figure 20). This indeed is a general principle when testing for strength. If a patient is reluctant to exert full power, then exert no resistance at all but encourage the patient to try, and when he or she does then one can suddenly increase the resistance. In this way one can encourage the patient to exert full power for a second or so, revealing normal strength. Obviously pain prevents full power being exerted and allowance must be made for this. Do not forget wasting is a feature of a lower motor neurone lesion and I find it useful to measure limb circumference, especially in the legs. More than 1 cm difference is significant, although of course there may be causes for wasting other than a lower motor neurone lesion. My version of the myotomes is shown in Table 1. Other authors may differ but I find my version works in practice.

Lack of facility as shown by asking the patient to 'play the piano' is a useful sign of an upper motor neurone lesion affecting the hands. This is

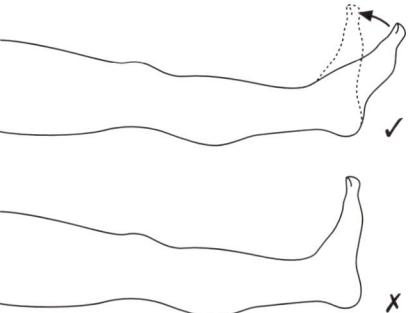

Fig. 20 It is vital to use the correct way to test the power of dorsiflexion of the foot. Most doctors have been incorrectly taught and this most important sign (of an L5 or S1 root compression) is missed. If the patient is asked to 'bend the foot back and keep it there' then the patient can lock the foot in that position and disguise an appreciable weakness.

present often before formal weakness is obvious. Testing for spasticity by sudden passive pronation–supination movement is also extremely helpful. Remember there is an upper motor neurone distribution of weakness, best remembered by recalling the hemiplegic posture, thus revealing movements such as shoulder adduction, elbow flexion, hip extension are stronger than the opposite movement. Therefore an upper motor neurone lesion will be first revealed by weakness of shoulder abduction and hip flexion.

Intracranial cause of footdrop

Most patients with a footdrop have an L5 root lesion, but not all. Sometimes a lesion arising from (meningioma) or near (glioma of the corpus callosum) the falx cerebri may present with a footdrop because the 'foot' part of the motor homunculus is sited there. Such lesions may cause diagnostic errors but there are two clues: usually the plantar response is extensor and often (but depending on the exact site of the lesion) there are no sensory symptoms or signs. Furthermore there is absolutely no pain, but sometimes one can see a relatively painless footdrop with an L5 root lesion. If in doubt scan the head!

Table 1 Myotomes.

Arms		
C5	Shoulder abduction	Deltoid reflex
C6	Elbow flexion	Biceps reflex
C7	Elbow extension	Triceps reflex
C8	Finger flexion	Finger flexion reflex
T1	Abductor pollicis brevis (median nerve)	
	Abductor digiti minimi (ulnar nerve)	
Legs		
All movements are L5 and S1 except:		
L2 and L3	Hip flexion	
L3 and L4	Knee extension	Knee or quadriceps reflex
L4 and L5	Inversion	
S1 and S2	Plantar flexion	Ankle reflex

L5 and S1 myotomes act at each joint, i.e.
Extension of hip
Flexion of knee
Dorsiflexion and eversion of the foot (and toes)

The ankle jerk differentiates between L5 and S1 because there is 'no L5' in the ankle reflex

Reflexes

The reflexes are particularly important as these do not rely on patient co-operation, except for the need for the patient to relax and have their attention diverted. What is often not appreciated is that you can hear an absent reflex. A dull thud with or without asking the patient to 'reinforce' by clenching their teeth or pulling their hands apart, signifies an absent reflex. I find this useful. Try it!

Using the reflexes one can cover most of the nerve roots of the lower cervical plexus. The deltoid jerk is useful but little known. Strictly it is a muscle reflex but by placing a finger on the deltoid insertion and hitting it with a reflex hammer, a reflex contraction of the deltoid muscles indicates an upper motor neurone lesion. The upper fibres of the trapezius may be used likewise, indicating a level above the C2/3 spinal cord level. An 'inverted' reflex is a useful sign. If one performs the biceps reflex and gets no response from the biceps reflex itself but finger flexion occurs instead, then this indicates a lesion at the C6 level of the spinal cord producing a lower motor neurone lesion at the C6 level and an upper motor neurone lesion at the C8 level (finger flexion). This is called an 'inverted biceps reflex'. These nuances are important because the clinical assessment of a patient with spondylotic radiculopathy or myelopathy is critical in determining treatment. The MRI scan assessment leaves a lot to be desired in elucidating these conditions.

I would ban all instruments of torture, such as keys, in the performance of the plantar response. Keys usually produce a flexor withdrawal response to pain. One must titrate the stimulus to the sensitivity of the patient's foot and start, with a thumb nail, on the outer border of the foot and work towards the sole of the foot. A true extensor plantar response does not occur until the thumb approaches the ball of the foot.

Sensory testing

One can be too obsessional when it comes to sensory testing and beginners often find areas of sensory loss that reflect no more than the natural variation of skin sensitivity, e.g. the lateral thigh is often less sensitive than other areas. When passing from a soft area to an area with underlying bone there is often enhancement of pin-prick sensation. I find the best way to test light touch is to rub the affected area and ask the patient to compare this with the normal. Often the patient comments that the act of rubbing produces a 'pins and needles' sensation. It is worth knowing that profound joint position sense loss produces 'pseudo-athetosis'. By this I mean when the patient holds his or her fingers outstretched with the eyes shut, the fingers move up and down in a random fashion due to a lack of feedback maintaining a still posture. If the patient claims to have no joint position sense of the fingers then absence of pseudo-athetosis would question how organic this loss is.

Of course *the* physical sign of spinal cord compression is a sensory level. If the patient is in coma, perhaps from a head injury, cord damage may be difficult to diagnose. Three signs are useful: a sweat level; retention of urine and 'warm shock'. Retention of urine is distinctly unusual in a head injury patient (incontinence is the rule) whereas the sympathectomy created by a cord lesion produces a dry, warm, vasodilated skin and hence the sweat level and a low blood pressure.

Dermatomes

The dermatomes are important to know. One does not need to remember the boundaries but the point of maximum sensation for any particular dermatome, i.e. the thumb for C6. C5 is over the point of the shoulder, C7 the middle finger, C8 the little finger, T1 is along the ulnar border of the forearm (this is where to look for sensory loss with a cervical rib) and T3 is in the axilla. Not many trainees realize that there are three fingers' breadth of C2 over the angle of the jaw. The leg dermatomes are well known, but what is less well known is that one needs to examine the pericoccygeal (not perianal) region for sensory loss with cauda equina compression. Sensory loss is first seen there and I have never seen a neurogenic bladder without pericoccygeal sensory loss, contrary to what some books state.

Cranial nerves

The main tip I pass on concerning the cranial nerves is when examining for a lower motor neurone facial weakness one must 'look for blinking'. Many books give long and convoluted advice to help decide if there is an upper or lower motor neurone facial weakness. It is really quite simple: look for a lack of or even a delayed blink. If this is present a lower motor neurone lesion is present and this is the earliest sign of such a weakness. Get used to watching how people blink!

I suppose the most commonly omitted cranial nerve sign (other than the sense of smell which has rather lost its importance with the advent of scanning, which reveals olfactory groove meningiomas so well) is the visual fields. How you examine these depends on the pathology. The earliest sign of chiasmal compression is a bitemporal scotomatous field loss. So place a red pin either side of the fixation point and ask the patient if there is a difference of redness on either side. An optic radiation lesion produces a homonymous hemi- or quadrantopia and this is first picked up by applying simultaneous stimuli to both visual fields. I remember well MacDonald Critchley holding a sixpence and a five pound note up in front of a patient (the note in the hemianopic visual field). He then exhorted the patient to 'take the money' in front of 200 trainees. Of course the patient took the sixpence and rumour has it that he always retrieved the sixpence from the patient later! If a patient is drowsy or obtunded then hold up both hands in each visual field and ask the patient to 'take my hands' and even quite drowsy patients will demonstrate their hemianopia in this fashion. Even less cooperative patients can be tested by 'menacing' either visual field and seeing if they blink or not. The visual fields are important, as the pathways travel through the temporal and parietal lobes en route to the occipital cortex. They cover a large area of the brain!

It is a useful manoeuvre to ask the patient to hold the arms out horizontally with the eyes shut. If there is weakness, the arms fall; if there is a cortical sensory loss the arms move up; if the arms move up and down a cerebellar loss is possible and if the fingers show pseudo-athetosis then there is a profound joint position sense loss. Instant neurological examination!

Other tips

Before leaving any patient it is obligatory to stand the patient up 'heel to toe' with the eyes open then shut. Truncal ataxia may be the only sign of a cerebellar vermis tumour and this is a particularly important test to do in children of course.

Remember there are three causes of a stiff neck: meningeal irritation, tonsillar herniation (coning) and something wrong with the neck. Limitation of straight leg raising may be due to meningeal irritation, nerve root compression (lumbar disc prolapse especially) or something wrong with the hip. Crossed straight leg raising is a wonderful physical sign; i.e. lifting the 'good' leg causes pain down the opposite leg. It is perhaps the most pathognomonic sign of a disc prolapse. I personally find the femoral stretch sign less helpful. Often the best way to assess straight leg raising is to watch the patient get on and off the couch. Most patients without true limitation of straight leg raising will sit transiently with their straightened legs at a right angle to their bodies when getting on the couch, and I find this a good informal method of assessing the true straight leg raising. Often patients with sciatica are 'conditioned' to have limited straight leg raising on formal testing. Another method is to ask the patient to sit up 'so I can examine your back'. Often patients with 'illness behaviour' are only too keen to do this whilst revealing an ability to perform a full straight leg raising to 90% with both legs.

A useful manoeuvre is to ask the patient to hop on either leg as this often brings out a latent weakness as does asking the patient to walk on their heels and toes. These tests come into their own if the patient for any reason is unable to fully cooperate with formal testing of strength.

I no longer examine patients for insurance companies but when I used to do this one needed a variety of examining techniques to flush out the non-organic signs. I remember a man with complete numbness of one leg as a result of an industrial injury. I examined him supine then rapidly turned him prone and stuck the pin in the 'numb' area. The change of position confused him and the single initial 'ouch' was his undoing. This I find more useful than the old chestnut of asking the patient to say 'yes' when you feel it and 'no' when you don't. Yet another patient hobbled in and out on crutches but a furtive glance at him walking down the road outside the hospital showed him walking easily, carrying the crutches under his arm.

chapter four

Making a diagnosis or an organized guess

A diagnosis is a guess but at least it ought to be an organized guess. There are books that describe how to take a history and examine the patient and those that describe the various pathologies. Yet how do you actually diagnose the pathological problems which are so minutely described? The answer is you need an intermediate phase. This seems one of the best kept secrets in clinical neurosurgery, but pathologies of the brain usually present with a combination of just three disorders: localized lesions (or multi-focal or diffuse), raised intracranial pressure (RICP) and meningeal irritation. Thus, the clinical features of intracranial disorders do not need to be individually learned but memorized in terms of focal lesions causing focal signs, RICP and meningeal irritation. This makes everything much easier and more organized! Actually, the same intermediate diagnostic phase can be used elsewhere. For instance, with intra-abdominal disorders one can decide if there is bowel obstruction, peritoneal irritation, free fluid or a lump before going on to make a pathological diagnosis.

An organized guess

Thus, an 'organized guess' is made in three phases, in order:
1 the structural and functional diagnosis;
2 the 'anatomical' diagnosis;
3 the pathological diagnosis.

Structural and functional diagnoses

Taking a history and carrying out an examination will define the disorders of structure and function. Neurology is mainly concerned with function but occasionally there are lumps on the head (and elsewhere) that need a diagnosis. Beware of the midline 'sebaceous cyst', it may be a dermoid cyst tracking into the posterior fossa! Sometimes the disorder may have no obvious anatomical or pathological basis such as migraine or epilepsy and the diagnostic process ends at this phase. It is at this stage the doctor decides if the weakness is due, for instance, to an upper motor neurone (UMN), a lower motor neurone (LMN) or a muscle disorder; or if the speech disorder is dysphasia or dysarthia, etc. Note that dysphasia is often misdiagnosed as confusion. Thus, the history and examination is used to elucidate the structural and functional disorders and then to define their exact type.

'Anatomical' diagnoses

There is a certain journalistic licence calling this group the 'anatomical' diagnosis but this is the all-important intermediate phase. From the earlier definition of structural and functional disorders one decides if there are focal neurological signs, RICP or meningeal irritation. Consideration of the focal signs will allow you to decide if there is a focal neurological lesion, which may be multi-focal or diffuse. One needs only fairly basic neuroanatomical knowledge to decide this and, as mentioned earlier, the examination tells you 'where the problem is' while the history more often tells you 'what the problem is', i.e. the pathological diagnosis. It is reassuring to know that if you cannot find, from history or examination, any features of focal signs, RICP or meningeal irritation, you are very unlikely to be missing anything serious at that particular time. It follows that you have to know all about RICP and meningeal irritation. These will be discussed later.

Pathological diagnoses

There are various pathological possibilities which in British medicine are enshrined in what is called the 'surgical sieve' (Table 2). I have no idea why it should be called a sieve and the disorders are not just 'surgical' but perhaps surgeons use it as opposed to physicians or 'internists'. How do you decide which of these runners is going to win the diagnostic race? Of course you consider the disorders of structure, function, the three possible 'anatomical' disorders, then consider the age, sex, speed of onset and subsequent course of the illness as well as the presence of disorders elsewhere, including any lumps in other parts of the body. Meningiomas occur in middle-aged women; the pathology of posterior fossa tumours is very age dependent. Medulloblastomas or cystic cerebellar astrocytomas occur in the first decade, while

Table 2 'Surgical sieve'.

Causes
Congenital
Traumatic
Inflammatory (or infective by viruses, bacteria or parasites)
Neoplastic (primary or secondary)
Vascular ('pipes blocked or burst')
Degenerative
Metabolic
Toxic

Which is the cause depends on:
Structural and functional diagnosis
The anatomical diagnosis (focal disorder, raised intracranial pressure and meningeal
    irritation)
The age and sex of the patient
The speed of onset and subsequent course
The presence of disorders elsewhere

haemangioblastomas occur in the second or third decade and metastases (usually presenting with vertigo for reasons I do not know) occur in the fifth decade onwards.

A simple example will illustrate use of this scheme. A patient with a headache, speech disorder and difficulty moving the right side will, on the first stage, be found to have dysphasia and an UMN lesion. The second phase will find (because papilloedema was found and the headache was worse at night-time) there is RICP. Furthermore, the focal signs suggest a lesion in the left frontal lobe. The third diagnostic phase considers the 'anatomical' diagnoses and decides the combination of focal signs, and RICP suggests a lump. The history is one of slow onset and progressive worsening over 6 months which suggests the lump is getting bigger. A 6-month history suggests a glioma but a short history of 1 or 2 weeks would indicate an abscess, a metastasis (if there is a known primary) or a high-grade glioma. A 1–2-year history, especially in a woman, suggests a meningioma whereas in some parts of the world a tuberculoma or parasitic infection might be more likely.

This scheme at least allows one's guess to be organized and the differential diagnosis to be logical. It also provides a way of organizing various disorders of the central nervous system, so it can be used for remembering the causes of, say, coma or epilepsy, etc.

Raised intracranial pressure

It is not my intention in this notebook to provide an exhaustive account of RICP. The features depend on the speed of onset: very rapidly increasing pressure causes coma whereas a slow increase causes dementia and an undue tendency to drop off to sleep at inappropriate times. The symptom is headache, worse in the morning or waking the patient at night. Headache in a comatose patient appears as restlessness and sweating. It is often said papilloedema is the most important sign of RICP. It is not. Drowsiness or decreasing conscious level is the most significant sign because papilloedema takes time to develop and may not be present despite serious RICP. Sudden RICP may cause retinal haemorrhages or even subhyaloid haemorrhages, seen on fundoscopy.

False localizing signs

False localizing signs are important. They arise due to distortion of the brain stem at the tentorial notch or foramen magnum (Figure 21). The features of brain-stem herniation at the tentorial notch depend on whether there is a lateral distortion (as occurs with an extradural haematoma) or vertical, downward distortion (as seen with bilateral subdural haematomata). Lateral distortion produces an ipsilateral third nerve palsy and only with extreme distortion, bilateral third nerve palsies. Displacement of the contralateral cerebral peduncle against the contralateral tentorial notch can produce an ipsilateral weakness which can be very confusing. For example, a patient with a right subdural haematoma may compress the left cerebral peduncle producing a right hemiparesis without the expected dysphasia in a right-handed person. Severe distortion may obstruct the posterior cerebral artery producing occipital lobe infarction and a hemianiopia (Figure 22). A patient of mine with a frontal lobe abscess recovered completely except for a hemomonous hemianopia. Of course, severe distortion damages the perforating arteries entering the brain stem producing decerebrate rigidity and, eventually, death. Bilateral extensor plantar responses occur early due to cerebral peduncular displacement.

Vertical downward displacement produces sixth nerve palsies because of the vertical course of these nerves, whereas lateral distortion affects the horizontally directed third nerves. In addition, downward displacement produces limitation of upward gaze, due, it is said, to distortion of the superior colliculi. I am not sure I believe this because the superior colliculi are well

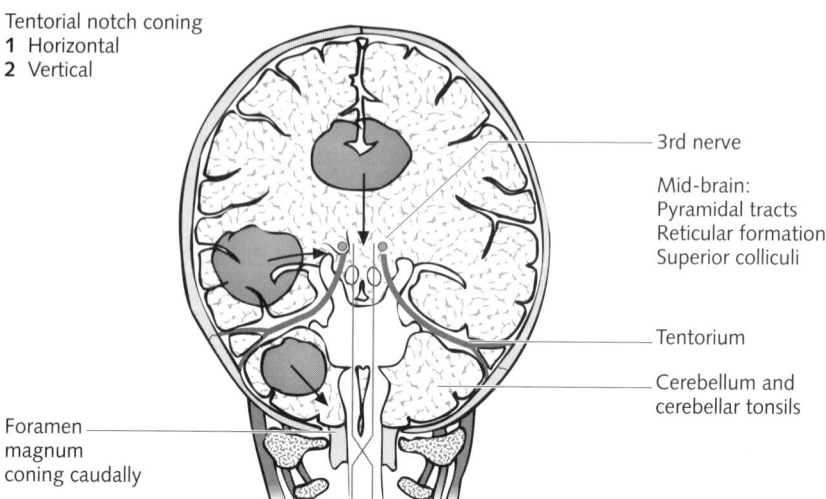

Tentorial notch coning
1 Horizontal
2 Vertical

3rd nerve

Mid-brain:
Pyramidal tracts
Reticular formation
Superior colliculi

Tentorium

Cerebellum and
cerebellar tonsils

Foramen
magnum
coning caudally

Fig. 21 Diagram to show the mechanism of 'false localizing signs'.

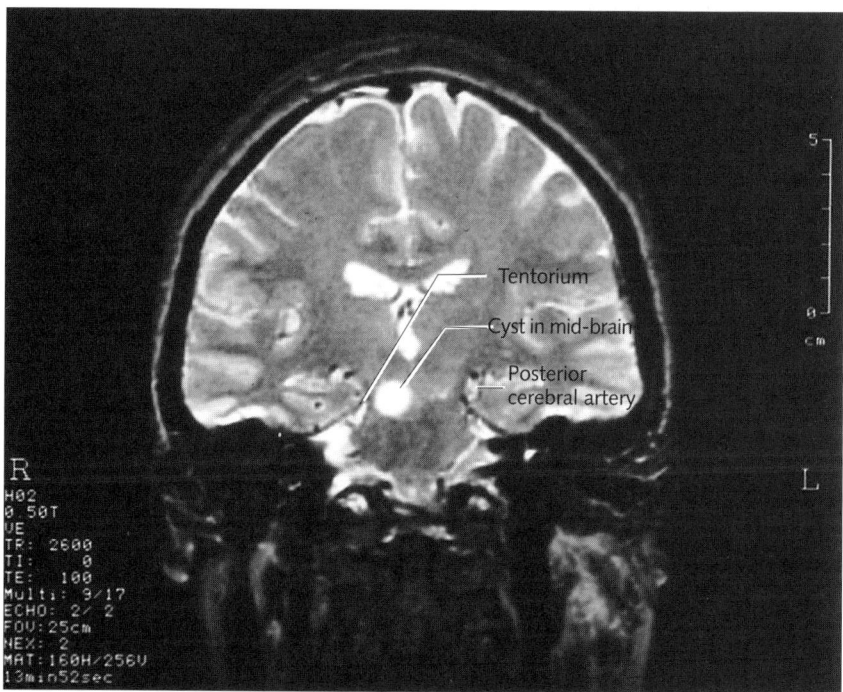

Tentorium

Cyst in mid-brain

Posterior
cerebral artery

Fig. 22 An MRI scan to show the posterior cerebral artery coursing around the mid-brain at the level of the free edge of the tentorium.

away from the tentorium but certainly limitation of upward gaze is a useful sign whatever the mechanism.

Coning

'Coning' is the name given to medullary compression by cerebellar tonsils in the presence of a posterior fossa tumour. The patient has a stiff neck (one of the three causes of a stiff neck) and stops breathing but maintains the circulation. The treatment is a burr hole to tap the enlarged ventricles and draw off cerebrospinal fluid (CSF). Its incidence has been much exaggerated and probably more people have died from meningitis due to a reluctance to do a lumbar puncture (for fear of coning) with consequent delay in diagnosing the meningitis, than have died from coning.

Causes (Figure 23)

The causes of RICP are summarized as:
1   too much CSF, called hydrocephalus;
2   too much pathological tissue;
3   too much blood, either arterial due to raised carbon dioxide levels in the blood or venous due to obstruction of venous outflow causing 'benign intracranial hypertension'; the final cause is the head being too small, i.e. craniosynostosis.

It is useful to consider causes of RICP without obvious focal signs, which is not an uncommon scenario. These include a right frontal (non-dominant) tumour, hydrocephalus due to obstruction of the ventricle (obstructive hydrocephalus, perhaps due to a colloid cyst or pineal tumour) or of the subarachnoid space (communicating hydrocephalus). Multiple small metastases, typically with a lot of surrounding oedema, may well present with RICP without focal signs and also a chronic subdural haematoma, especially if bilateral, and especially in the not so elderly, may do the same. Finally, 'benign' intracranial hypertension may cause frighteningly severe papilloedema, with little headache. It is not benign because it may cause blindness. One is allowed an extensor plantar and a sixth nerve palsy, but anything more negates this diagnosis and suggests instead a diffuse infiltrating glioma; some gliomas infiltrate and expand both cerebral hemispheres and brain stem with remarkably few focal signs.

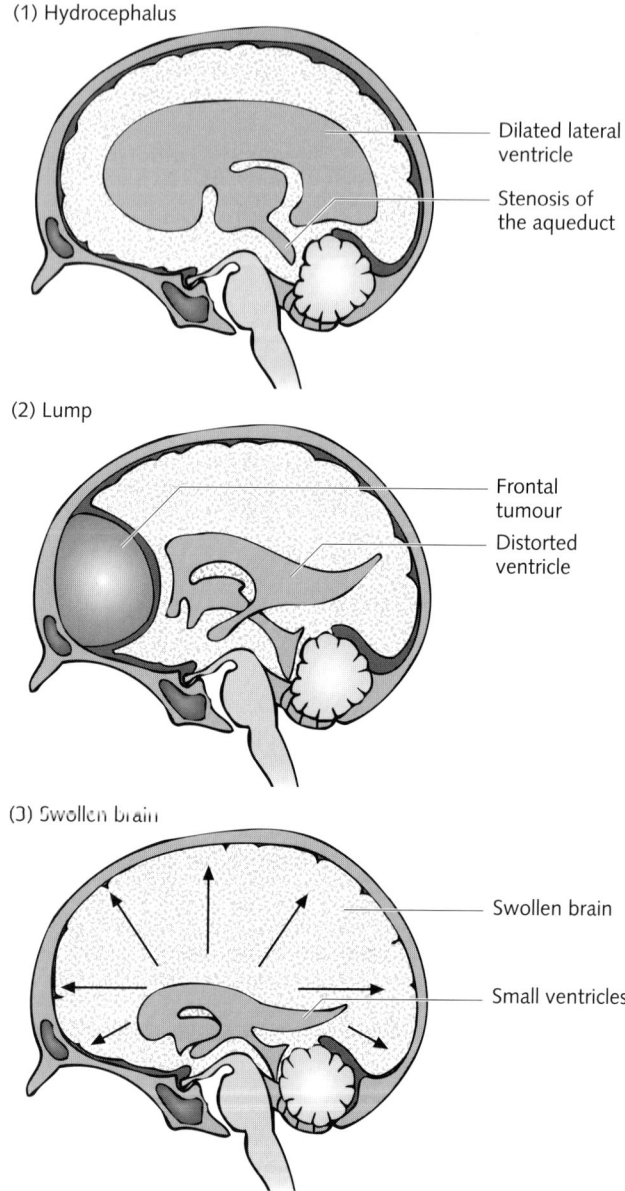

(1) Hydrocephalus

Dilated lateral ventricle

Stenosis of the aqueduct

(2) Lump

Frontal tumour

Distorted ventricle

(3) Swollen brain

Swollen brain

Small ventricles

Fig. 23 The three causes of RICP.

Meningeal irritation

Causes

The features are well known, but why photophobia is so much a feature of meningeal irritation as opposed to RICP, I have no idea. The causes of meningeal irritation are the same as pleural or peritoneal irritation. These are:
1 blood (a sudden unusual headache lasting more than 24 hours means a subarachnoid haemorrhage until proved otherwise);
2 pus (you need 24 hours of life left to treat meningitis so do that lumbar puncture this evening rather than tomorrow morning);
3 chemicals (drugs introduced by doctors into the subarachnoid space or occasionally cholesterol from a craniopharyngioma or epidermoid cyst); and finally
4 cancer cells, either glioma or carcinoma cells.

Investigation

If the symptoms and signs indicate meningeal irritation, the only way to decide the cause is to do a lumbar puncture. There is an increasing trend to diagnose subarachnoid haemorrhage using the CT scan. There are two disadvantages to this: first, the patient with the smallest bleed, who is the very best patient for the surgeon, may have insufficient blood to show on a CT scan (these patients comprise about 15% of the total); secondly, the diagnosis of meningitis may be delayed if the physician does a CT scan, a test done only during the daytime in many hospitals and not in the evening when many of these patients are admitted.

The indication for a lumbar puncture is therefore meningeal irritation; the contra-indication is a posterior fossa mass causing RICP. Note, not all causes of RICP are contra-indications for a lumbar puncture. Indeed, communicating hydrocephalus is well treated by repeated lumbar punctures.

Focal signs

Before we leave this chapter it is perhaps worth mentioning that meningiomas, for their size, produce fewer focal signs than gliomas. Thus, an occipital mass without a hemianopic field loss on examination is much more likely to be a meningioma than a glioma, which is much more likely to produce a visual field loss. This was well known to a past generation of neurosurgeons but the advent of scans coupled with the (regrettable) decline of clinical assessment has meant these sort of facts have been forgotten.

There are two last points. When assessing an MRI scan for hydrocephalus look at the temporal horns. The lateral and third ventricles may remain dilated even after the pressure has been reduced but the temporal horns are the best guide. Secondly, always look at the optic fundi (as well as the MRI scan) in patients with hydrocephalus; I have seen severe papilloedema and progressive visual failure in these patients with remarkably normal-looking scans—even normal-looking temporal horns!

One patient was unique in my experience: a young man had a ventriculo-peritoneal shunt inserted at another hospital for aqueduct stenosis. Since that day he had had abdominal pain and headache. We converted the shunt to an atrial shunt which cured his abdominal pain immediately. We attempted to cure the headache, which was due to over-drainage (slit ventricles), by inserting a programmable shunt. This initially failed to prevent over-drainage until we had, in addition, introduced an anti-syphon device and 'fine tuned' the pressure. We found that 130 mm was too little and he had 'over-drainage' headache (and slit ventricles) and 140 mm was too much and he had hydrocephalus (and large ventricles). I was amazed at just how precise a pressure was needed. I debated about introducing a more finely tuned programmable shunt which the manufacturers kindly offered to make, but in the end I advised an old-fashioned operation: a Torkildsen's procedure passing tubes from the lateral ventricles to the cisterna magna, thus obviating the need for any external shunt system. I had not previously realized that the correct shunt pressure might need to be so precise, nor that CSF in the peritoneum could cause such pain.

It is worth remembering an old-fashioned operation for aqueduct stenosis: a posterior fossa decompression may allow the aqueduct to dilate up. I had one patient with aqueduct stenosis who was very shunt dependent, lapsing into coma whenever the shunt malfunctioned. I performed a posterior fossa decompression and since that day she has had no further trouble.

By the way, I must mention 'normal-pressure' hydrocephalus. Actually it is, of course, intermittently raised pressure. Some neurologists do not believe it exists, so I recount this story of one patient of mine. He was (and is) a successful businessman. When I first saw him he had mild ataxia, dementia and incontinence. There was no antecedent history of meningeal irritation, i.e. subarachnoid blood or infection. He saw two senior neurologists; one did not believe in normal-pressure hydrocephalus and the other thought he had cerebrovascular disease. I did a lumbar puncture to draw off CSF. His timed walking distance improved after the lumbar puncture but he declined the offer of a shunt. Later his family took him abroad and he was told a shunt was too risky. I next saw him 15 months later. The aggressive, dominating man had become passive, withdrawn, wheelchair bound and doubly incontinent. He had retired from business. It was with considerable reluctance that his family then agreed to a shunt operation. A Codman programmable shunt was inserted (he was on warfarin and was diabetic, hypertensive and obese) and after reducing the pressure from 180 to 120 he started to improve. Within 2 months he was back to his normal aggressive self. He got rid of his wheelchair and reinstated himself at the helm of his business. One suspects that not all members of his family were quite as delighted about this dramatic change as the patient was. Yes, normal-pressure hydrocephalus exists but yes, it can be hard to diagnose, especially if there is no antecedent history of meningeal irritation. But to miss the diagnosis is a tragedy. I do find 'therapeutic test lumbar punctures' about the best test; I am unhappy to monitor the intracranial pressure and so risk infection being introduced. I would advise that 'if in doubt, shunt' but use a programmable shunt, because such shunts reduce the risks of subdural effusion and, should one occur, allow its treatment in the least traumatic fashion; one still has to let out the effusion but the shunt can be easily turned off and on, moreover at different opening pressures.

chapter five

A few fundamental general surgical principles

You may ask why I should include some general surgical principles in a neurosurgical notebook. I do so for three reasons. The first is that knowledge of these principles makes sense of the art and craft of surgery; secondly, when I need to retreat to basic principles to unravel a problem, I am grateful to know them; and thirdly, I never perform an operation without thinking of at least some of these principles even though I have been operating for over 30 years.

As a young man I was intensely frustrated reading a textbook of surgery. There seemed no thread or science. One learned a chapter on abdominal surgery then an apparently quite separate chapter on urogenital surgery, etc. Different chapters, different problems and different solutions. I then realized that this was incorrect and that apparently different surgical specialities were all concerned with similar tissues and similar problems using similar surgical principles. Neurosurgery, like other types of surgery, is involved with repairing trauma, removing lumps, stopping haemorrhage, dealing with diverticula, eliminating abscesses and infection, relieving obstruction, diverting fistulae, excising sinuses, curing ulcers and improving, if possible, function. I then discovered that if one looked at different chapters each speciality dealt with, for instance, diverticula and the causes of diverticula are similar, as are the complications and indeed the principles of treatment. Suddenly, and with a degree of excitement that I can still recall today, I realized that there was a thread or a series of threads, throughout surgery, and suddenly the whole thing made sense. How much easier I would have found surgery as a student if some book or somebody had told me this sooner!

Lumps

I have no intention of reproducing the contents of a basic textbook of surgery and I will assume the reader knows the mechanics of examining a lump (Table 3). Of course a history is taken, then a physical examination, the purpose of which is to try and define first the precise anatomical position of the lump and secondly the characteristics, especially concerning the contents of the lump. This is of course done by inspection, palpation and auscultation, with due regard to the surrounding or adjacent structures such as the lymph glands, nerves and blood vessels. One then has the problem of how to make a diagnosis, or organized guess. Once again the textbooks describe how to examine the lump and then describe the various and many lumps in considerable detail without helping the trainee to decide which lump is which. So one needs an intermediate phase just as one does for diagnosing intracranial problems.

Table 3 Lumps.

1 Examination of a lump

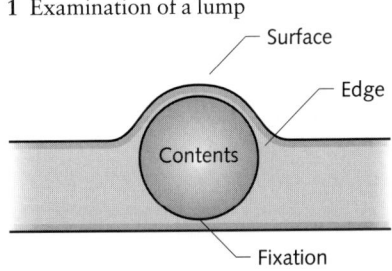

2 History	? pain, ? speed of growth
Inspection	Situation, shape, size, surface—colour
Palpation	Tender, temperature
	Surface, edge, fixed to skin or muscle, etc.
	Contents
	Consistency
	Fluctuation in two planes
	Trans-illumination
	Expansile pulsation
	Cough impulse
	Reducible
	Change of consistency with position
Auscultation	? bruit, ? fixed to skin or deep structure

3 Types of lumps—four types
Acute inflammatory
Cystic
Diverticula
Solid

How to diagnose a lump

A lump is diagnosed in three phases. The first is to obtain the facts concerning the structure and function by taking a history and performing an examination. The second stage is to decide from the facts obtained at the first stage, which of the four types of lump this represents, i.e. inflammatory, cystic, diverticular or solid. An inflammatory lump has the signs of Celsus (but be aware that infarction or a tumour such as a sarcoma may mimic an inflammatory lump, being painful, tender and possibly hot). A cyst (and usually the signs will indicate a soft cyst because a tense cyst will not be distinguishable from a solid lump), will have the features of fluctuation in two planes and possibly trans-illumination, if the cyst fluid is clear.

A diverticulum characteristically shows two features, first expansile pulsation either on coughing or during arterial systole and secondly reducibility. Expansile pulsation has to be differentiated from transmitted pulsation (on coughing or systole), which implies the lump is adjacent to a structure that expands on coughing or systole but is not part of such a structure. There may also be an alteration of consistency with change of posture implying a venous diverticulum. Of course a bruit, or turbulence, may be heard on auscultation during systole, which implies either a sudden change of vessel diameter and/or fluid velocity. A bruit that extends into diastole means a flow of blood even during diastole, which in practice indicates an arteriovenous fistula of some type.

Having decided which of these subgroups the lump is, one can decide on the basis of the lump's anatomical position and attachments, as well as the history and the possible pathology. Once again the process becomes a logical guess, and a reasonable differential diagnosis suggests itself. Of course lumps do arise on the head and therefore this scheme is of practical value to the neurosurgeon.

Diverticula

Diverticula exist in all parts of the body from hernias, bladder diverticula, Meckel's diverticula, aneurysms, meningocele and encephaloceles. Their aetiology is either congenital or acquired and if acquired they arise either because of a weak wall or an increase of intraluminal pressure, or both. The treatment may be excision, strengthening the wall or reducing intraluminal pressure, or, again, both. Thus, the treatment of an intracranial aneurysm may be excision (especially a mycotic aneurysm), strengthening the wall (wrapping), eliminating the intraluminal pressure by excluding the aneurysm from the circulation with a clip on the neck of the aneurysm or by thrombogenic coils introduced by the endovascular route. Hunterian ligation is still used to reduce the flow to an aneurysm by reducing the intraluminal pressure; typically this is used for a giant basilar trunk aneurysm in neurosurgery.

The cause of saccular aneurysms is as yet unknown but certainly there is an increased incidence in children with coarctation of the aorta inducing hypertension. Atheroma (and in former days, syphilis) causes fusiform aneurysms by weakening the wall, usually of the basilar artery (Table 4).

Infection

Infection may occur due to general or local factors and it is the local factors that are of profound importance to the surgeon. These factors determine surgical technique and it is these that I never fail to think of when I carry out any operation. The factors are listed in Table 5, which also describes the necessary techniques to avoid these factors. In addition to these predisposing factors one has to consider the source of infection. All wounds

Table 4 Diverticula.

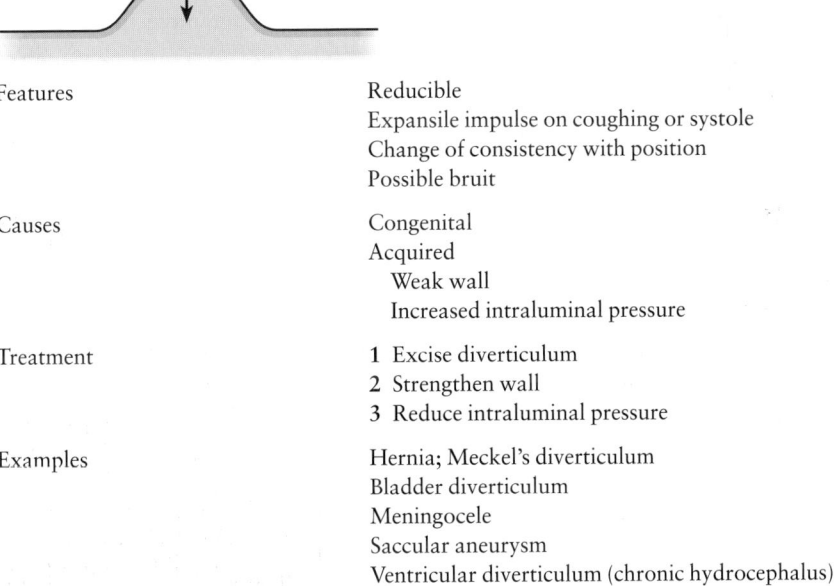

Features	Reducible Expansile impulse on coughing or systole Change of consistency with position Possible bruit

Causes	Congenital
	Acquired
	    Weak wall
	    Increased intraluminal pressure

Treatment	1 Excise diverticulum 2 Strengthen wall 3 Reduce intraluminal pressure
Examples	Hernia; Meckel's diverticulum Bladder diverticulum Meningocele Saccular aneurysm Ventricular diverticulum (chronic hydrocephalus)

Table 5 Predisposing factors for local infection and how to avoid them when operating.

Haematoma	Careful haemostasis
Dead space	Careful closure in layers; use a suction drain
Dead tissue	Avoid excessive diathermy or ligating large amounts of tissue; remove necrotic bone, often a cause of a persistent post-operative sinus
Ischaemic tissue	Avoid excessive retraction; gentle operative technique
Foreign body	Avoid black silk sutures etc.
Undue contamination	Avoid excessively long operations; avoid skin contamination by covering skin edges and discourage the assistant from excessive 'wiping' during closure

become contaminated but clearly the shorter time the wound is open the less contamination occurs. A quick, yet unhurried, operation is desirable. Secondly, too little attention is paid to the skin edges, as these are frequent sources of, for instance, shunt infection. I cover the edges with iodine-soaked swabs and discourage my assistant from wiping the edges whilst sewing up, pointing out the likelihood of *Staphylococcus epidermidis* being swept into the wound during this much loved manoeuvre by the assistant (Table 5).

I now give all my patients prophylactic antibiotics and have no doubt this reduces infection. I base this confident statement on the virtual elimination of that most unpleasant condition called 'discitis' following lumbar disc surgery by using a single dose of peri-operative antibiotic.

Abscess

The causes, features, complications and methods of treating an abscess are the same throughout the body and so if one understands the principles, these can be applied to any abscess. The cause is either locally introduced or spread by way of the blood stream from a source elsewhere. An abscess is essentially a bag of pus and the wall of the bag is initially granulation tissue. After about 6 weeks fibrinous tissue starts to become fibrous and by definition an abscess surrounded by fibrous tissue is more completely walled off, and in these circumstances it is more feasible to excise. The principles of treatment are to wall off the infection with antibiotics and remove the pus. In an examination candidates are expected to say they would obtain a sample of pus before starting antibiotics. In practice a general cocktail of antibiotics is started immediately pre-operatively, pus obtained later and the antibiotics modified once the organism and its sensitivities have been discovered. There are three ways to remove pus: drainage, aspiration or excision. Drains are sometimes used for subdural abscesses but it is my experience that a generous craniotomy and excision of the abscess, especially the otherwise not easily reached parafalcine component, gives much better results. Aspiration is the usual method for an intracerebral abscess and I advocate daily aspiration to empty the abscess and ensure it remains empty. Excision of an intracerebral abscess is performed if aspiration fails, either because of a foreign body within the abscess, a thick wall or a multi-loculated abscess not satisfactorily drained by aspiration. The old textbooks advocate excising cerebellar abscesses because of the danger of rapidly developing obstructive hydrocephalus. Cerebellar abscess has become a remarkably rare lesion in my practice nowadays.

With any abscess, but particularly a brain abscess, it is important to treat the cause, such as sinusitis, middle ear disease or congenital cyanotic heart disease, as well as the complications. Epilepsy is common and anticonvulsants are needed. RICP is a particular feature, not just due to the amount of pus but also to the degree of surrounding oedema, which is a characteristic of brain abscess. If RICP is severe then steroids are life saving but of course steroids should only be used once the diagnosis is established. Ventriculitis or rupture of the abscess into the ventricle is a devastating complication and usually fatal. Although the MRI scan appearance usually suggests the diagnosis, I have operated on one woman with an 'obvious glioblastoma' on the MRI that turned out to be an abscess (Figure 24). This is a good reason for biopsying most if not all 'glioblastoma multiforme'. Another patient of mine with a past history of an astrocytoma causing hydrocephalus and requiring a ventriculoperitoneal shunt, was refused admission to the neurosurgical unit that put in the shunt because he had a 'recurrent tumour'. In fact he had a temporal lobe abscess which occurred a few months after appendicitis and the infection tracked into the head via the shunt, from the abdomen.

Fistula

A fistula is an abnormal communication between two epithelial or endothelial lined surfaces. It may be congenital or acquired. The most important principle of treatment is that a fistula will be maintained as long as there is persistent distal obstruction. The commonest intracranial fistula is an

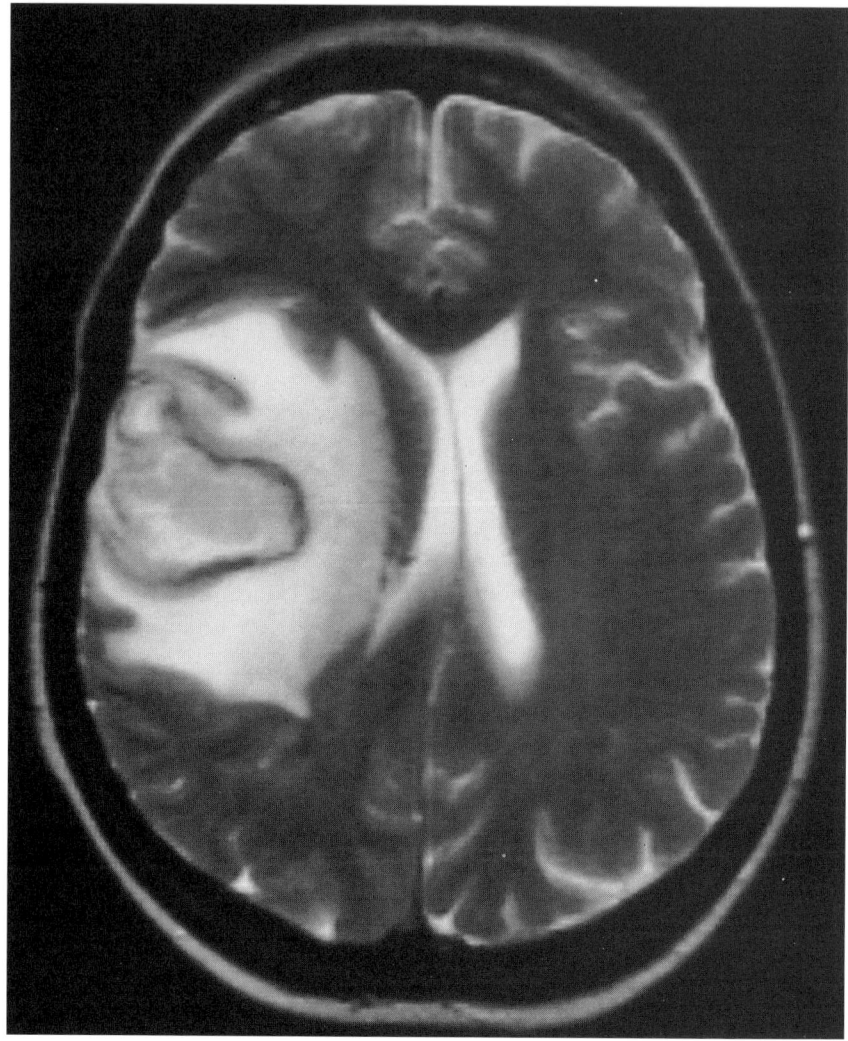

(a)

Fig. 24 (a,b) MRI scans of a 'typical glioma' that turned out to be an abscess. (*Continued*)

arteriovenous malformation of the brain or dura. Traumatic arteriovenous fistulae occur such as a caroticocavernous or vertebral–venous, the latter occurring after surgery in the vicinity of the vertebral artery (or in past days, radiologists attempting percutaneous puncture of the vertebral artery). In these circumstances treatment is directed to occluding the fistula.

CSF fistulae are also common and one does have to be sure there is no distal obstruction (such as a communicating hydrocephalus) in order

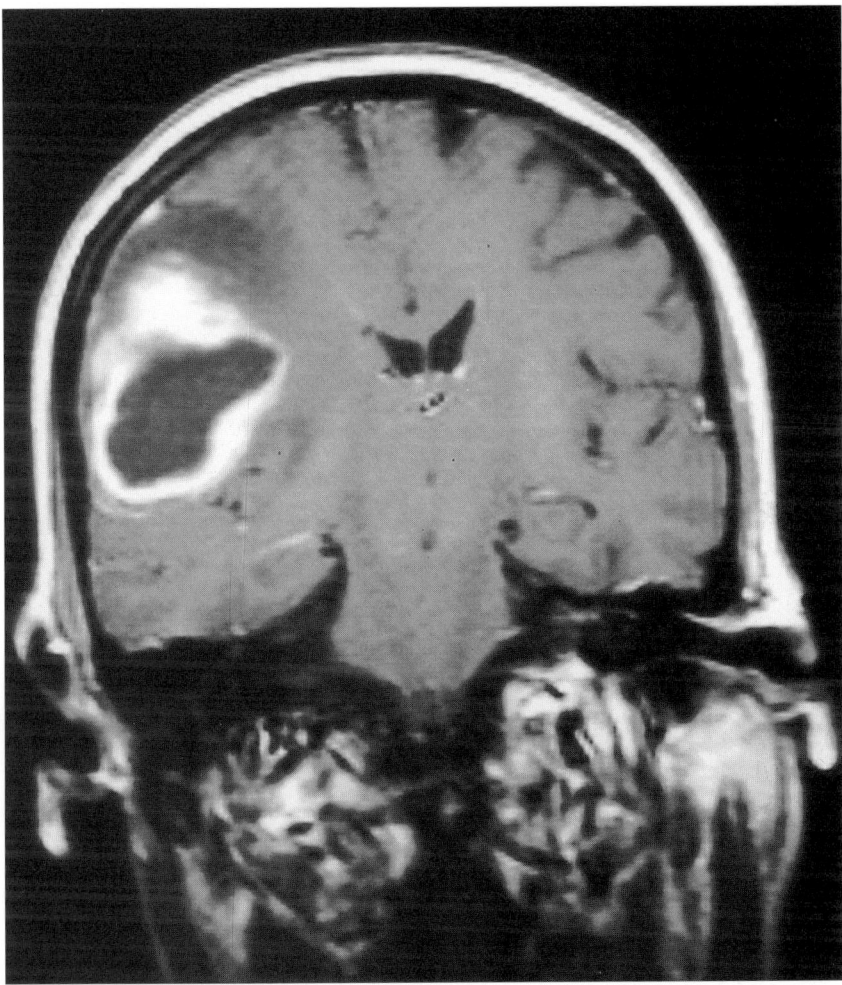

(b)

Fig. 24 (*Continued*)

to successfully stop the CSF leak. Thus, persistent leakage of CSF through a wound may be due to one of two causes. The first is that a communicating hydrocephalus has developed, either because of intraoperative release of blood or post-operative infection (i.e. meningitis), and until this 'distal obstruction' is relieved, the leak of CSF will persist (see Table 6 and Figure 25). The second cause is a small hole in the arachnoid. Small holes, as opposed to big holes, cause a great deal of trouble in surgery because they act as one-way valves, allowing CSF out during moments of

Table 6 Fistula.

Causes	Congenital
	Acquired
	Trauma
	Inflammatory
	Neoplastic
	Infection
Treatment	1 Treat any infection
	2 Relieve the distal obstruction
	3 Excise or obstruct the abnormal communication

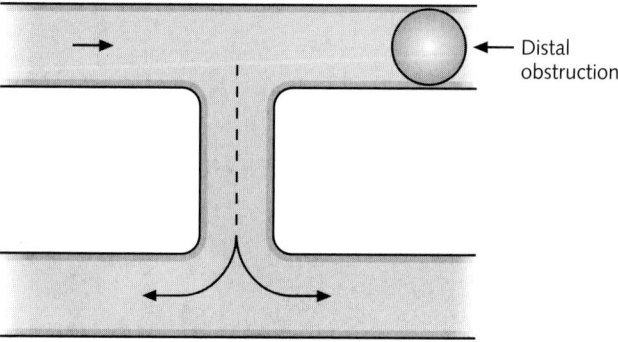

Fig. 25 Diagram to emphasize the importance of relieving any distal obstruction when attempting to eliminate a fistula.

RICP (coughing, straining) but do not allow its return (as does a large hole). Thus, CSF builds up under high pressure, eventually leaking out. The cure is to repair the hole or alternatively, open the arachnoid widely to destroy the 'valve'.

chapter six

Talking with patients

I could have entitled this chapter 'talking to patients' but I hope when you have read it you will see why I didn't. Before we discuss talking with patients we must talk about you. Yes you—and me. I have a highly intelligent daughter who has taught me so much. She taught herself to read and spell at the age of 4 and she happens to have that mysterious condition called dyspraxia. She communicates with us by typing, or touching letters on a board. She has a photographic memory, profound wisdom and insight. She has a highly developed sense of intuition and knows how someone feels inside themselves. She has taught me that if I am physically with her but thinking about what I have done, or have not done, or need to do, then she knows it and is unimpressed. Other people, and that means patients, are exactly the same; they know if you are giving them 100% of your attention and if you are not, they too are unimpressed. You will find you do not necessarily need to spend a long time with patients as long as when you are physically with them you are 100% attending to them. This process is helped if you sit down near them and listen as well as talk and when you talk, remember the KISS principle!

One of the best kept secrets of life

Let me tell you one of the best kept secrets of life. I took a long time to learn it and wish I had known it earlier. However much you think you disguise your feelings, thoughts and prejudices—you don't! In other words it is glaringly obvious to other people (yes, patients!) how you feel internally. If you are tense, unsure, miserable, worried and unsympathetic, the patient will know and respond fairly negatively. The patient will be unique if he or she is not tense, unsure, miserable and worried talking to a neurosurgeon. I became a consultant (specialist) neurosurgeon at Oxford at the age of 32. At the age of 35 I was head of the department, conscious of its past reputation, anxious to introduce new ideas and technologies. I found myself performing operations I had not seen or done before with no one to turn to for advice. There were no scans in those days to make our lives, and the patients' lives, easier. How was I to my trainees? I was difficult, demanding and distant. I hope they realized I was doing my best for them and my patients, but I was really wearing a badge saying 'I am young, inexperienced and worried!'. It is said that over the years 'he mellowed'. I certainly became more confident and more relaxed having seen and done a lot more surgery.

The message is this: all patients, without exception, are anxious. Sometimes they are 'difficult' (i.e. very anxious) and even abusive (extremely anxious). Sometimes you may feel you do not actually like a patient. The best way to deal with people and therefore patients and indeed colleagues as well as your trainees, is to approach them with a feeling of warmth for them. You may have to look for and even dig for some aspect of a person's personality which you find warming, but this you must do. I recommend this to you for not only will it help your patient (or colleague or trainee or indeed anyone else) it will actually make your own life much more enjoyable.

Empathy

One quality that is needed is 'empathy'. I suppose by empathy I mean the ability to fully understand the concerns of that particular patient. Every doctor likes to feel he or she has empathy but not all do. Empathy does not just depend on being sensitive oneself but it first depends on receiving information, often unconsciously, from the patient. Close observation of patients will provide a lot of information. How they greet you, how they hold themselves (body language), how they talk, etc.

Whether relatives are in attendance may be quite informative. Being warm and paying complete attention to the patient will demonstrate a concerned and interested doctor with whom the patient can have confidence in and confide in. It never ceases to amaze me how often patients say what they really mean just as they are walking out of the door! The best way to learn empathy is to be a patient oneself and spend time in hospital, or to be a parent of an ill child. Alternatively, watching a good doctor and learning by example is extremely helpful, but some people have to work harder than others to learn empathy.

There are various times when one communicates with patients: the first time one sees the patient and discusses the diagnosis and treatment; prior to the operation you come into contact with the patient to consent them; and finally one sees the patient after the operation. Taking a history necessarily involves a great deal of communication and it helps to spend time putting the patient at ease, being empathetic as well as a good listener. The next stage is to discuss the possible problems and which tests you feel are appropriate. Simplicity, i.e. clarity of thought, expressing what you think the problem is and why you think it is, gives the patient much confidence. After the investigations it is necessary to discuss the treatment with the patient. I never tell the patient to have an operation. I describe the problem to the patient as clearly and simply as I can, never stating beyond what is really known. If the patient has a brain tumour, perhaps a glioma, I will say there is a swelling or lump and the only way to ascertain its nature is to take a piece to examine under a microscope. I avoid speculating if at all possible at this stage even though the patient often wants you to speculate. If excision is contemplated then one can say it might be possible to remove some of it, or all of it at operation, depending on what one finds. You can point out that if nothing is done the likelihood is that the patient will get worse. When the problem is pain, such as sciatica, then it is even more necessary to give the patient options between operation and conservative treatment. I describe as factually as possible the advantages and disadvantages of either course of treatment and what an operation would entail. I then stress that the operation is to stop pain and that only the patient can decide how much the pain affects his or her life. The time to have surgery is when the patient realizes that he or she has had enough of the pain. Thus, it is a psychological decision and this varies from patient to patient. The surgeon may obtain some impression of the severity or otherwise of the pain but only the patient can make the decision about what to do.

Consent

It is incumbent on the surgeon to discuss risks so the patient has 'informed consent'. How informed the consent is varies considerably. Some patients surf the Internet for information while others implore you not to give them any more information. When discussing risk it is important not to frighten patients, and the concept of informed consent implies that a balanced, sensible assessment of risk must be given to the patient so that the hoped for benefits can be weighed against the risks of surgery as well as the risks of not operating. In other words, the natural history of a disorder without treatment must also be discussed. This exercise is especially important in neurosurgery where the margin for error is often smaller than in other specialities and the effects of brain damage are profound for the patient and, indeed, the relatives. Most patients have an understandable fear of being left intellectually damaged should a complication occur. It is a good rule never to persuade a patient to have surgery, however convinced you are of the need. Patients have a right to decide their own fates and if the patient decides he or she does not wish the surgeon to open the head and remove a convexity meningioma, then so be it. You can be sure that persuading or coercing a patient to have surgery will almost certainly result in that patient developing complications! I sometimes think the unusually anxious patient, perhaps because of a high noradrenaline level, is unusually liable to develop complications whereas the confident, calmer patient is much more likely to have a smoother post-operative course.

The risks

I have a fairly standard approach to discussing risks of operation. I first describe the risks of any operation, i.e. the anaesthetic, a blood clot and infection. I point out that if these occur in the brain the consequences are often more serious. I then discuss the specific complications of the particular operation. These subdivide into (almost) inevitable, possible or rare but devastating complications. For example, a temporal lobectomy will be likely to produce an upper quadrantic visual field loss. In the UK, this would disallow the patient to drive and this must be explained. If the meningioma is abutting the internal carotid artery then a risk (I usually quote 2–3%) of a 'stroke' occurring must be mentioned. The risk of facial weakness after removal of an acoustic neuroma depends, of course, on the size of the tumour, but in these circumstances I describe the three possible outcomes: a normal functioning face, temporary paralysis of the face with complete or incomplete recovery, or severing the nerve and the need to carry out a nerve graft procedure. I make a point of actually mentioning that the eye will not close and the mouth will droop because patients do not really understand what 'a facial weakness' means if it happens to them.

Discussing the risks that exist with every operation is, I think, one of the most difficult tasks for a surgeon. Much of this interchange needs empathy, sensitivity, simplicity, clarity of thought and expression, and careful choice of words. Saying too much may confuse, yet too little will be unhelpful. A diagram often helps. Occasionally, a simple bald statement such as 'the risks of surgery are less than the risks of doing nothing', if it is appropriate, is helpful; for instance in the situation of a patient with a ruptured intracranial aneurysm. It is important to state in the notes or in a letter the nature of the risks that have been discussed with the patient and a percentage chance of such risks developing if percentages have been given.

The patient must also understand that the surgeon may be unable to decide what can and cannot be done until the time of the operation. The difficult problem of judgement will be discussed later but the patient does have to understand that the pre-operative investigations do not always accurately prophesy the anatomical and pathological situation that will confront the surgeon.

A little touch of Harry in the night

I always make a point of seeing patients before I operate to remind me of salient features, such as which is the side of the pain or the side of the paralysis. At this time I encourage the patient and promise that I will do my very best. Of course you will, but it does help the patient to hear this from the surgeon, for the operation is probably the single most important event of his or her life. 'A little touch of Harry in the night' was the way Shakespeare described how Henry V went around the tents of his outnumbered army the night before the Battle of Agincourt. The operation will be a battle for the patient (and the surgeon) and I recommend 'a little touch of Harry in the night', especially before a major intracranial procedure.

After the operation

Following the surgery the patient needs to be told about the operative findings and what was done and not done as well as the prospects for recovery or otherwise. There are two practical situations which a neurosurgeon has to deal with. First, the patient may have quite marked neurological deficits even after, or perhaps especially after, a benign tumour such as a meningioma has been removed. Patients and indeed non-neurologically trained doctors have little understanding of the remarkable powers of recovery of the brain. A useful rule is that 70% of recovery that is going to occur, occurs in the first 6 months and the other 30% in the following 18 months. Indeed, I removed a ruptured arteriovenous malformation in a paediatric cardiologist. This was in the left frontal lobe and caused aphasia and a profound right hemiparesis at the time of the bleed. Two years later he was back at work performing cardiac catheterizations on babies, yet he told me that he was so appalled by his initial deficits that he saved up his sleeping tablets with a view to killing himself. I have found it useful to know that the hand and speech 'go together'. If someone is aphasic but the hand is moving then speech is likely to recover, and vice versa. The second common problem is a glioma.

Glioma

A problem that confronts the neurosurgeon all too often is the need to explain to the patient and relatives about a glioma. I first explain it is not a tumour that usually spreads to other parts of the body so in that respect it is not a cancer. I find the simplest way to explain the pathology is to ask the relatives (and/or the patient) to imagine the brain to be a bowl of white paint into which a blob of red paint (glioma) has been introduced. Three zones are produced: a red zone of pure tumour, which the surgeon can safely remove; a pink zone comprising tumour and brain mixed together, which the surgeon cannot safely remove or indeed recognize with certainty even with an operating microscope—this zone can only be treated with radiotherapy; and a zone of normal brain. I go on to say that the amount of 'red' and 'pink' varies from tumour to tumour; sometimes there will be no red zone and on other (rare) occasions little or no pink zone. Using this simplistic but reasonably accurate model, patients and relatives have been able to understand the problem of treating these tumours.

As a trainee I was taught to be conservative in the management of gliomas. I am now either much more aggressive or I do the minimum, i.e. a biopsy. Surgical efforts between these two extremes in my experience are unhelpful and more likely to lead to post-operative complications of swelling or haemorrhage. I am convinced that the best palliation occurs from a radical removal of the tumour (i.e. the 'red' zone) followed by radiotherapy. The surgeon should not worry unduly about bleeding from the tumour vessels for this bleeding will miraculously stop once all the obvious tumour has been removed. It is important not to leave behind the 'purplish' tumour for this often swells or bleeds in the post-operative period. Either do a complete macroscopic removal or do the minimum but do not do something in between, which I refer to as 'tip and run' to use a cricketing metaphor. If in doubt though, at least do a biopsy. Figure 24 (pp. 56–57) shows a 'typical glioma' on the magnetic resonance imaging scan that turned out to be an abscess.

Complications

Complications inevitably occur. Usually these have been discussed pre-operatively but occasionally a complication occurs that is distressingly unexpected. Pulmonary embolism is the commonest but I have had four patients who developed haemorrhagic cerebellar infarction after contralateral frontal craniotomies for benign lesions such as meningiomas or aneurysms. The operations all went particularly well and took very little time. No one could foretell such a complication. Undoubtedly the best policy is to be extremely frank and honest with the relatives at all times. Nothing engenders a lack of trust and confidence more than a feeling that the surgeon may be less than frank and open. It is an interesting quirk of human nature how difficult it can be to enter the room and explain and re-explain why and how the complication may have arisen and what the outcome may be. Failure to do so only adds to the relatives' distress and ultimately damages the bond of confidence that hopefully has been built up. Certainly, to express sorrow that a complication has occurred is in my view only right and does not mean you accept any legal liability.

Bad news

Giving bad news to the patient is never easy. I am frequently appalled by how insensitively it can be given. I learned by example as a young doctor how one can tell a patient he or she may not live long without being frightening. 'The pathologist has seen a few cells which are growing rather more rapidly than he would like and therefore I cannot guarantee the future. If you have any arrangements you feel you should make then I suggest that would be sensible'. This tells the patient all he or she needs to know. It is truthful and accurate. I have invariably used this form of words. Avoid statements as to how long someone has to live. For a start, prophesying a time is almost certainly going to be inaccurate and secondly, I believe it is extremely important to leave the patient with some hope, especially in the initial stages of the illness. If one studies any series of patients with glioblastoma multiforme there are always a few who survive much longer than expected. Statistics can only reflect the average and they are meaningless for the individual.

There does inevitably come a time when it is clear the patient is going to die. At this stage pain relief, loving care and dignity are needed. Time for bereavement that starts before death is necessary. Too often the other side of medicine is all too easily forgotten in these days of high technology. We cannot always cure; all of us have to die and a part of medicine just as important as performing difficult and complex surgery is to allow patients to die free of pain, with dignity, surrounded by loving care.

The most stressful part of neurosurgery

Personally I find the most stressful part of neurosurgery is to provide emotional support to the patient and relatives in the post-operative phase during which slow, but hopefully gradual, recovery of neurological function is occurring. It is at this stage that the patient's confidence in the surgeon is paramount. One needs to be confident in one's own predictions and to be able to express these predictions sensibly. One has to be caring, understanding, prepared to discuss time and time again questions and problems. I find it helpful to explain that the only way a doctor can predict the future is to draw a graph in his or her mind's eye. If there is improvement each week then the graph is likely to continue to show an upward curve, whereas a horizontal line suggests little likelihood of improvement, and a descending line, of course, deterioration. This aspect of neurosurgery is very demanding yet so little is written about it. Of course the operation must be done with as much skill and judgement that the surgeon can muster but no good surgeon can confine him- or herself to operative work and ignore the much more demanding, emotionally wearing and lengthy post-operative phase, restoring self confidence and belief of the patient and his or her family.

This process can be made much easier for everybody if the pre-operative communication has engendered a strong degree of trust and confidence. These aspects of surgery certainly demonstrate the personal qualities of the surgeon, perhaps even more so than his or her behaviour in the operating theatre.

chapter seven

When to operate, when not to operate and when to stop

This chapter concerns judgement, and judgement is the single most important attribute for a surgeon. Just because an operation is possible, it does not mean it is right to perform such an operation. A surgeon without judgement is a danger, yet it is remarkable that so little is written about this considering its importance. Perhaps this is so because it is not an easy subject upon which to write and so much is learned at the trainer's elbow. I will make some general observations. Young neurosurgeons tend to over-operate. Tired surgeons certainly over-operate because it is easier to say 'operate' than 'let us wait and see'. Perhaps the most difficult thing of all is to know when to stop during the operation. If one can do this then one has probably learned surgical judgement. It is a remarkably difficult thing to do, as emotionally the surgeon feels he or she ought to complete what the patient has been promised.

When to operate and when not to operate

I have found it useful to consider three major factors (Table 7).

The patient has to be 'right'

By this I mean the age, general health and outlook have to be reasonable. What is 'reasonable'? I am loathe to have strict criteria for age, for in general I prefer to try and assess the number of years from the grave rather than from birth. We all know some people of 70 can be remarkably fit and spry yet others of the same age can be particularly old and infirm. Clearly the general health is crucial; whether the patient is an arteriopath, on anticoagulation or perhaps has a known malignancy elsewhere are all crucial factors. Yet do guard against rigid guidelines and I have never understood why some

Table 7 When to operate and when not to operate.

The patient has to be 'right'
The brain (or spinal cord) has to be 'right'
The lesion has to be 'right'. This depends on:
    Clinical features from the history and examination
    The *anatomy* of the lesion and the anatomy of the access
    The *pathology* of the lesion
    The *natural history* of the lesion without operation
    The *relevance* of the lesion to the clinical features
    The *wishes* of the patient (and relatives)

---

neurosurgeons refuse to consider surgical treatment of subarachnoid haemorrhage for patients over the age of 65.

The brain has to be 'right'

To take one extreme example, there is no point operating on a particular pathology if the patient is brain-stem dead. Equally, if the patient is profoundly demented from perhaps a bifrontal glioma and yet the patient has no features of raised intracranial pressure, then one should be very circumspect about how much surgical treatment to advise. Another common situation is the patient who has had a severe intracerebral haemorrhage from an arteriovenous malformation or a severe subarachnoid haemorrhage from a ruptured aneurysm. Most of us have learned that emergency surgery has little advantage in these circumstances and it is much better to wait, and allow the patient, and the brain, time to recover. Often quite remarkable recovery can occur and then the pathology can be treated with a much better outcome than could have been envisaged earlier.

The only time when surgery is helpful is if the patient continues to deteriorate after the initial event. In these circumstances emergency surgery is often useful, because the deterioration may well be due to increasing raised intracranial pressure from obstructive hydrocephalus, or, much less frequently, expansion of the haematoma from continued bleeding. The key is in the history not the scan! For instance, one patient of mine, a doctor, felt dizzy and then collapsed and when found by his professional partner, the patient was able to utter a few words at that stage. Within an hour the patient was in coma. Clearly some pathology other than the ictal event was causing the progressive deterioration of conscious level. We evacuated the posterior fossa haematoma and later clipped the peripheral posterior inferior cerebellar artery aneurysm. The management of this patient depended on knowing he spoke after the collapse.

Sometimes it is possible to admit a patient after a bleed very quickly, perform angiography and take the patient to the operating theatre, evacuate the haematoma and excise the underlying arteriovenous malformation. One patient of mine, a young American girl staying in Oxford, bled at 1.00 pm on a Sunday and by 3.00 pm that afternoon she was in the operating theatre, a large haematoma was excised, together with the underlying arteriovenous malformation. She made a remarkable recovery even though by the time we took her to the operating theatre she had deteriorated markedly.

Other patients with a ruptured arteriovenous malformation are unfortunately brain-stem dead within a few minutes of the ictus and in these circumstances surgical intervention is of no use. Patients with ruptured intracranial aneurysms who suffer a respiratory arrest do not recover in my experience unless they have a ruptured posterior circulation aneurysm, particularly, for instance, a posterior inferior cerebellar artery aneurysm.

Just occasionally patients are put on ventilators after a subarachnoid haemorrhage without an actual respiratory arrest occurring and one has to be careful to differentiate this from patients who have had a true respiratory arrest following a subarachnoid haemorrhage. Once again rigid rules (or 'principles') should be avoided. I find it difficult to understand why some children are denied surgical treatment for epilepsy because of a low 'IQ'. Surely if surgery is likely to stop or significantly reduce the epilepsy then that child should be offered it irrespective of the IQ. Why should a child with a low IQ be denied surgery? These children may well show an improvement in the IQ after successful surgery for the epilepsy, but even if this does not happen surely it is better for a child to have just one problem rather than two?

The lesion has to be 'right'

Attention to detail is the most important factor in determining surgical judgement. In the end it is what you can achieve, not what a world-famous neurosurgeon claims he or she can (or maybe cannot) achieve. The surgeon has to decide whether a lesion can be removed without permanent harm to the patient. To assess the chances of success the surgeon needs to consider the six factors listed in Table 7.

Clinical features

The history is of crucial importance but it is of special importance in these circumstances. Careful attention to the chronological development of the symptoms and signs will often tell the surgeon where the lesion first arose, which may well be of particular help in assessing the operability of the lesion. It will also help when discussing the risks of the proposed operation with the patient. Furthermore, when removing a meningioma, reconstruction of the way the tumour has grown can be extremely helpful in knowing how to deliver the tumour. For example, when operating on a posterior fossa meningioma, to know if the tumour has originated from the under-surface of the tentorium and grown down so depressing the fifth, seventh and eighth nerves will allow the surgeon to deliver the tumour from below, upwards with much less damage to these cranial nerves.

The anatomy of the lesion and the approach

The second factor is a detailed knowledge and assessment of the anatomy. This perhaps is the most important factor of all and I still spend a long time examining the MRI scan, the 'bone window' CT scans and the angiograms, and then check details in anatomical textbooks until I have built up in my own mind a detailed picture of the anatomy. I cannot over-emphasize the importance of this. I certainly regret not doing this if I mistakenly think a lesion is a straightforward one, but I have never regretted the many hours I have spent thinking about the anatomy and going over and over it. Nowhere is this more true than in dealing with arteriovenous malformations. I always have a plan, which starts with planning an adequate exposure, planning which veins to use to lead me to the lesion and which arterial input to obliterate first. My operations do not always go to plan but at least I have a plan just as a general has a detailed plan before going into battle. But just as a general may have to alter his plans, so may the surgeon.

The surgeon's appreciation of the anatomy is not confined to the anatomical boundaries of the lesion but also, critically, towards considering which of the possible various approaches might be the best for removing the lesion with the least morbidity. For example, a cavernous angioma which has bled into the left cerebral peduncle of the mid-brain might be approached subtemporally but not without risk to the vein of Labbé. Would a trans-temporal pole approach be more appropriate or a trans-Sylvian (as for Yasargil's amygdalohippocampectomy approach) or even a trans-callosal trans-third ventricular approach be more appropriate? Possibly a posterior approach, a supracerebellar subtentorial approach may be the right one. Only detailed knowledge of the anatomy of the lesion, careful consideration of the anatomy of the approach (and some experience of the difficulties and dangers of each approach) combined with appreciation of the pathology (i.e. is it intrinsic, extrinsic, exophytic, well defined or infiltrative) will all be needed before the surgeon can properly advise the patient.

The pathology

A detailed appreciation of the extent and nature of the pathology is part of the anatomical assessment. Of course if one is dealing with a glioblastoma, the surgeon will not usually attempt a complete excision of the lesion but will stay within the confines of the tumour. But when faced with a suprasellar meningioma then careful assessment of the extent of the lesion and its relationships to the circle of Willis, cranial nerves and pituitary stalk will all need consideration. These can be appreciated pre-operatively by careful assessment of the MRI scan and the surgeon needs to have this 'picture' in mind when planning the operation. Indeed, without this the surgeon cannot discuss the specific risks of the operation with the patient.

The natural history of the lesion

Before one can conclude whether an operation is advisable, the surgeon must have some idea of the natural history of the disease. This may be difficult to assess without benefit of a histological diagnosis and this should be pointed out to the patient and the relatives. Usually, however, the surgeon may obtain a very reasonable idea of the biological activity of the tumour by ascertaining the length of the history to date, i.e. by taking a careful history from the patient. Of course, one has to differentiate what might appear to be rapid growth from a slow-growing tumour that has suddenly caused hydrocephalus or initiated epilepsy. The natural history of a ruptured aneurysm is now well established but for unruptured aneurysms, less so. What advice does one give a patient with a basilar trunk aneurysm that has not bled? Given the difficulties of access this may not be easy and requires careful consideration of all these various aspects that have been so far discussed.

Arteriovenous malformations pose great difficulties for the surgeon when considering the natural history. The size of a lesion is not helpful, indeed large arteriovenous malformations often do not seem to bleed as much as smaller ones, presumably because these would not have grown to a large size without bleeding if they had a propensity to bleed! There are figures for bleeding rates depending on previous bleeds, the presence or absence of epilepsy, neurological signs (not due to a prior bleed), etc. Often these lesions 'leak' rather than bleed catastrophically and often the patient may experience several bleeds and not be unduly incapacitated. This makes consideration of the natural history of intracerebral arteriovenous malformations perhaps the most difficult of all lesions that the surgeon has to deal with. Indeed it is impossible for the surgeon to be sure that an arteriovenous malformation will not bleed and so if it is possible to remove such a lesion safely, then it is better to do so.

When discussing the natural history with a patient it is important to emphasize as well the natural history following surgery; deterioration may be stopped but actual recovery takes time, being a function of nature, not of the operation. In some circumstances (such as meningioma surgery) the patient may be made worse by the operation only to improve or recover completely over the following 6 months or more.

The relevance of the lesion to the clinical features

Two other factors are important in the pre-operative assessment. The first is to be certain that the lesion demonstrated on investigation is indeed the cause of the patient's symptoms and signs. This is especially important in the spine where modern methods of investigation may reveal osteophytes and disc protrusions that are not the cause of the patient's complaints. Clearly, to operate in these circumstances is bound to produce a failed operation and a disappointed patient. The tendency to operate on scans and not on patients is increasingly prevalent due to the sophistication of modern imaging. Just occasionally similar difficulties may arise with intracranial lesions; for instance is the meningioma demonstrated on the scan the cause of the patient's 'transient stroke'? Does the mild and perhaps doubtful communicating hydrocephalus account for the patient's dementia?

The wishes of the patient

Last but certainly not least, one must take into account the patient's wishes. The role of the surgeon today is very much to give the patient options, to describe what each option entails, and their advantages and disadvantages. This is especially true when advising a patient with pain such as sciatica, because only the patient knows how severe the pain is and how much it affects his or her life. Indeed, the decision to opt for an operation is a psychological one, based on emotion, not logic and this may vary from patient to patient. When advising a patient with sciatica about the options, i.e. operation or conservative treatment, it is incumbent on the surgeon to consider the patient as a whole. Are there other factors? Is there undue depression? Is there a claim against an employer? Has the pain become a prop or a friend to the patient giving the care and attention he or she would not otherwise receive from the family? Is the patient addicted to analgesics? Equally the surgeon must emphasize that in general nerve root compression pain responds well to an operation but nobody can give the patient a new back. So if back pain is a predominant symptom, the surgeon should point this out.

Some patients will adamantly refuse an operation, however obvious its need is to the surgeon. This is their right and it should, indeed must, be respected. It is most unwise to persuade a patient to have surgery for it will be that patient that experiences complications. Equally, the surgeon should avoid the emotive statement that if the patient was his or her relative then the surgeon would have no doubt about advising an operation. I also refuse to answer the question 'what would you do?'. I point out that I am not the patient, that everyone is different and then repeat the options and the various factors to be taken into consideration. At this stage you might ask yourself if you would operate on the cavernous angioma in Figure 26(a,b). If so, how?

Operative surgical judgement

Surgical judgement is also required during the operation. This perhaps requires more finely tuned judgement than at any other time and the sign of mature surgical judgement is when a surgeon decides to stop the operation. This is more difficult than it might appear, as the surgeon has to battle with his or her own psychology. The surgeon will have advised the operation and will have the patient's and relatives' confidence. The theatre team will be prepared for perhaps a long and difficult operation. The surgeon will not want to admit defeat and lose face. All these factors must be put aside and instead the surgeon must ask him- or herself if the anatomy and pathology of the lesion have presented difficulties not apparent pre-operatively and the continuation of the operation will be more likely to do more harm than good.

Of course, during any operation difficulties will be encountered and these need to be overcome. One must therefore not 'give up' too easily. These difficulties must be contrasted with the situation where the surgeon finds the difficulties gradually mount up. I find one useful question to ask myself is

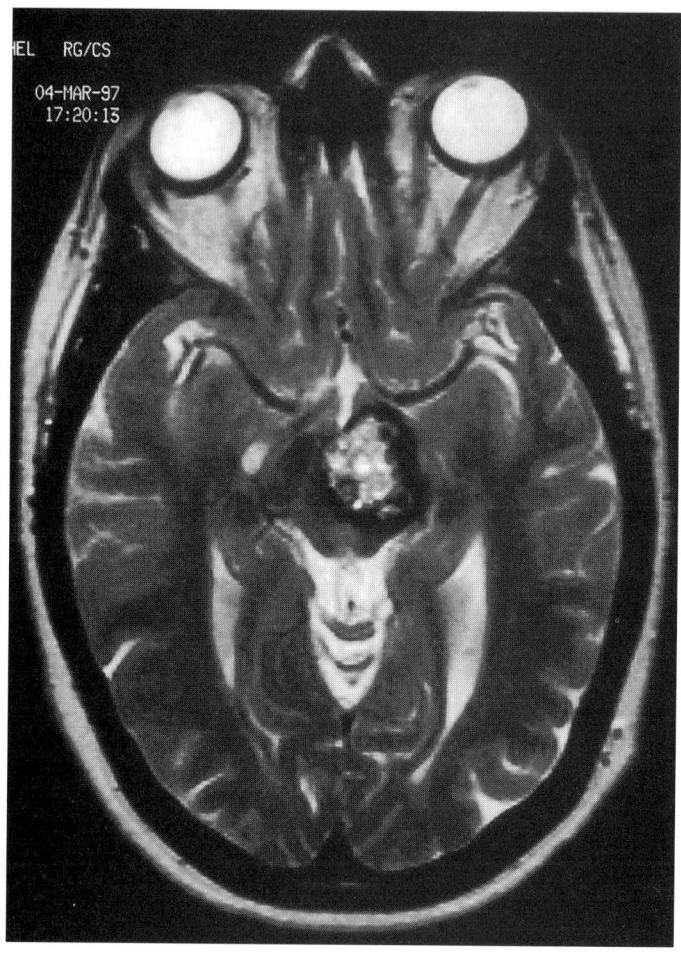

(a)

Fig. 26 (a,b) Would you advise surgery for this mid-brain cavernous angioma? If so, how? The patient, aged 40, was having increasing difficulty using her (dominant) right hand together with increasing dysarthria, but was able to lead an otherwise normal life without restriction. This lesion is in the peduncle affecting motor function of the right limbs and almost certainly affecting the optic tract and almost certainly will be near the third nerve nucleus. The posterior cerebral artery (and anterior choroidal artery and basal vein of Rosenthal) run over the surface of the lesion. (*Continued*)

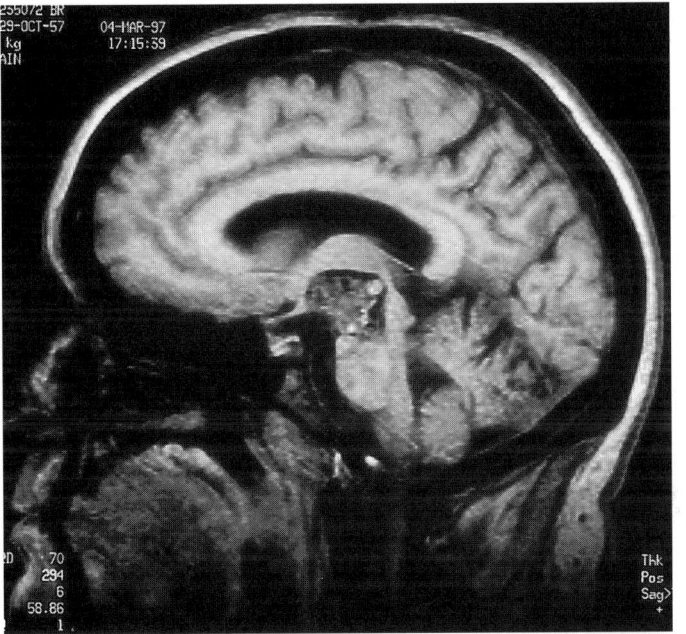

(b)

Fig. 26 (*Continued*)

this: 'am I going to be able to completely remove this tumour?' If the answer is apparently 'no' then clearly to take undue risks or produce severe morbidity in achieving a partial removal is unjustified. This situation is frequently encountered during an operation for a cavernous sinus meningioma. Is it sensible to cause an ophthalmoplegia if only 95% of the tumour can be removed when perhaps 80% removal of the tumour can be achieved without an ophthalmoplegia? The advent of stereotactic radiosurgery as a probably effective method for dealing with the remnant, crystallizes this debate. It is worth remembering that one can always come back another time if the patient is undamaged yet one can never undo severe operative brain damage. But this decision is never easy, as the surgeon knows that the first operation is the best time to achieve surgical excision. Nor is there an easy answer as to when and whether the surgeon should be bold or show discretion. Often the difficult operation one worries about turns out to be much easier, yet other 'easy' operations that have not produced too much pre-operative concern (perhaps due to misjudgement) turn out to be much more difficult. By the way, did you decide to operate on the mid-brain cavernous angioma in Figure 26? See Figure 26(c).

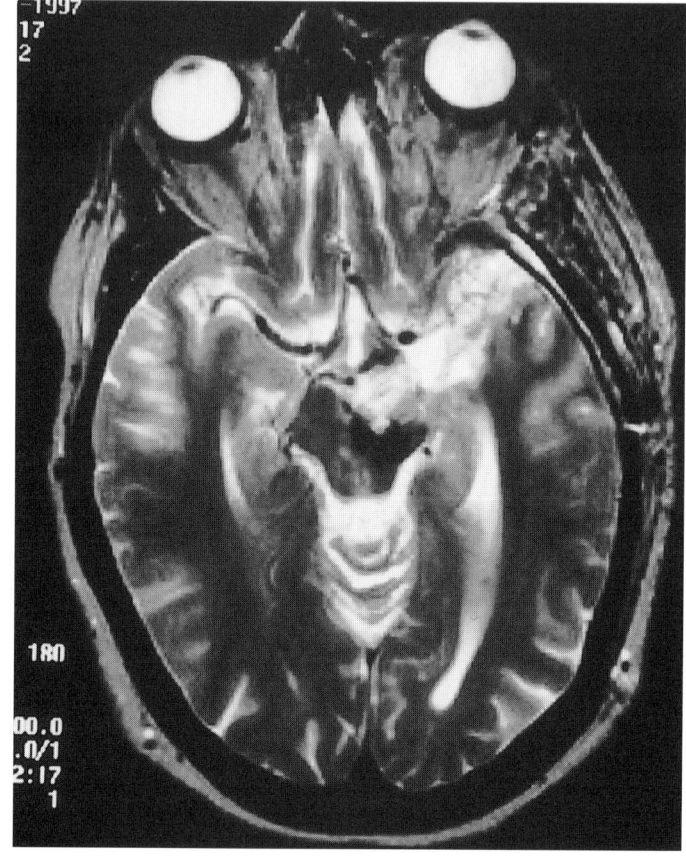

(c)

Fig. 26 (*Continued*) (c) The natural history of cavernous angioma is frequent bleeds. This one had bled, as shown by the black ring of haemosiderin. In the brain stem these lesions in my experience cause progressive and devastating disability. Once the surgeon has obtained access then they are usually not too difficult to remove, being like a blackberry with slow 'venous' flow. I advised surgery at this stage when the symptoms were beginning to be intrusive hoping that after surgery she would regain her pre-operative state, which would allow a near-normal lifestyle. I approached this through trans-temporal approach as for a basilar aneurysm. The optic tract had to be sacrificed but the third nerve was spared. The right hemiparesis was initially worse but she eventually made a good recovery and was spared the fate of progressive deterioration and probable death from recurrent bleeds.

Surgical judgement both before and during the operation represents the most sublime development of the surgeon. Lay people dwell on the surgeon's manipulative skill but it is judgement that is the major demand imposed on the surgeon and that is what, in the end, we are paid for and upon which our reputations stand or fall.

chapter eight

Some puzzling pathologies

There are three conditions that deserve to be better known. I do not pretend to understand them but knowing that they exist has helped me in my clinical practice. Curiously, they have received little attention in standard textbooks.

Translucent membranes and the central nervous system

Arachnoid cysts

Congenital

For many years I have been fascinated by congenital arachnoid cysts. Most commonly they occur in the region of the temporal pole, yet I have seen these intracerebrally often adjacent to the lateral ventricle. The temporal lobe cysts are often associated with an absence or failure of the pole of the temporal lobe to develop. Draining veins are usually stretched over the superficial surface of the cyst and the danger of such a cyst is the propensity of these draining veins to rupture and bleed after minor trauma. The interest, however, for me is the tendency for these cysts to expand the overlying bone, thus causing a visible bulging of the temple. Other arachnoid cysts expand, such as those within the cerebral hemispheres and I have seen these simple benign cysts misdiagnosed as cystic gliomas.

Acquired

I can record another similar lesion but of traumatic rather than congenital origin. In 1967, at the age of 31, this woman underwent a right frontal craniotomy for a pituitary tumour. She made an excellent recovery but in January 1979 developed severe generalized headaches, which persisted. In May 1979 she was referred to me. She was hypopituitary following

77

the pituitary surgery but had no other neurological signs. A CT scan (Figure 27) showed a large right frontal cyst displacing the right frontal horn. A metrizamide encephalogram demonstrated metrizamide in both lateral ventricles but the cyst adjacent to the right frontal horn did not fill.

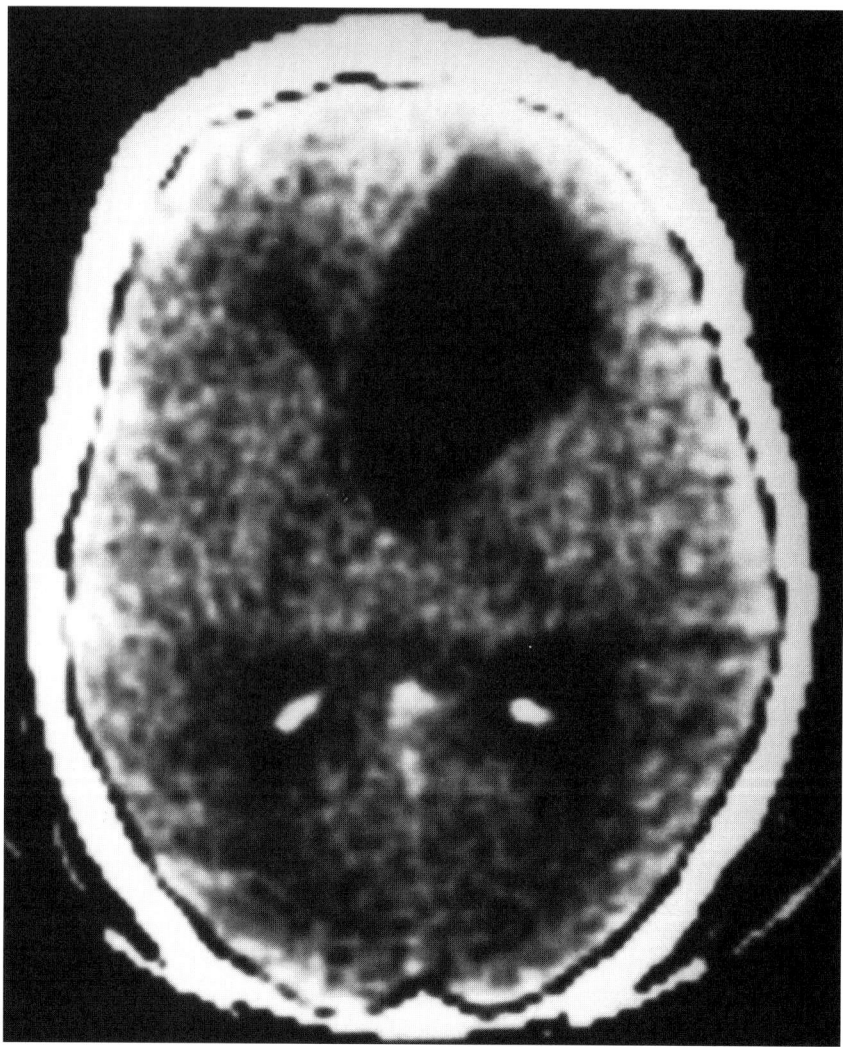

Fig. 27 CT scan to show the cyst extending between the subfrontal subarachnoid space and the frontal horn of the lateral ventricle, the cyst being created after pituitary tumour surgery.

On 17 May 1979, a small right frontal craniotomy was carried out. Through a cortical incision the cyst was entered. Clear, slightly yellow fluid was found. Inspection of the cyst wall showed no choroid plexus. Medially and inferiorly the cyst wall was separated from the subarachnoid space by a translucent membrane. Posteriorly the cyst was separated from the frontal horn of the right lateral ventricle by another translucent membrane. This was excised thus opening the cyst into the lateral ventricle. She made an immediate and complete recovery and was cured of her headache.

It seems likely to me that a small area of necrosis of the right frontal lobe developed during the retraction at the time of the operation for the pituitary adenoma. This area of necrosis was presumably immediately adjacent to the pia mater and the subarachnoid space. I surmised that a small cyst developed, which progressively enlarged until it was sufficient to cause severe headache and displacement of the adjacent structures. Drainage into the lateral ventricle cured her symptoms.

Traumatic syringomyelia

I will describe another patient in whom I have found translucent membranes adjacent to the subarachnoid space. This patient developed traumatic syringomyelia. In 1968, at the age of 30, this male patient crashed during a motorbike race. He sustained a fracture dislocation at T4/5 with complete and immediate paraplegia. In February 1977 (9 years later), he noticed weakness of both arms, especially the right, together with a change of feeling of both arms and hands. This weakness severely affected his ability to manoeuvre himself in his wheelchair. In September 1977 he was admitted to the Radcliffe Infirmary where weakness was noticed on shoulder abduction, flexion and extension at the elbow on both sides but more so on the right. There was wasting and weakness of the small hand muscles. A myelogram showed distension of the spinal cord, without herniation of the cerebellar tonsils, and the diagnosis of post-traumatic syringomyelia was made (Figure 28).

At operation on 9 September 1977, a cervical laminectomy from C3 to C7 was carried out. On opening the dura, the cord appeared distended and blue. A fine needle was inserted into the lower part of the syrinx and 2.5 ml of dark yellow fluid aspirated (protein content 5.2 g/litre). The lower part of the syrinx collapsed. As the upper, cranial, portion of the syrinx remained, this area was also aspirated and 4 ml of rather paler yellow fluid (protein 3.5 g/litre) was obtained. After this the collapsed dorsal part of the cord measured 3 mm across whereas the ventral part of the cord was normal in

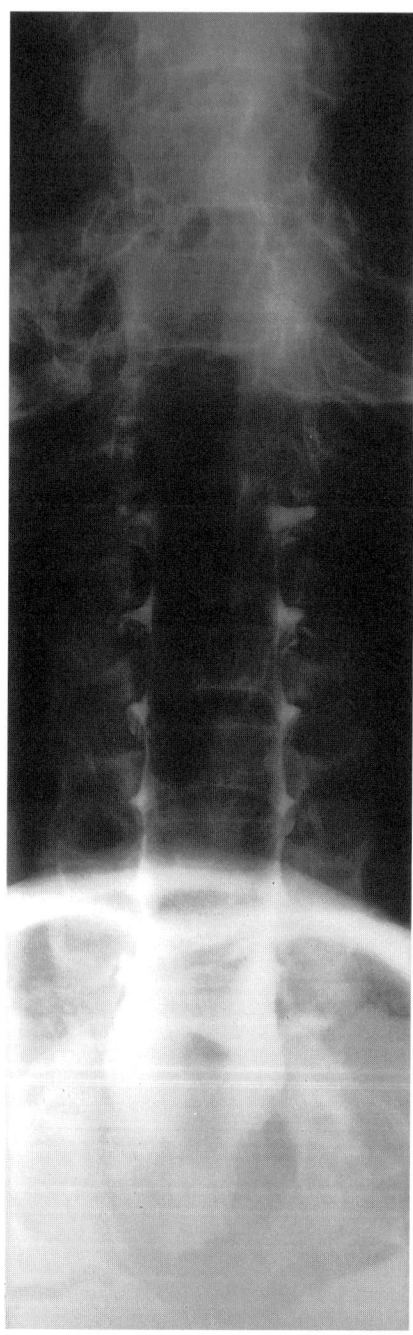

Fig. 28 Myelogram to show the swollen cord (so-called candle grease appearance) due to traumatic syringomyelia.

size. The middle part of the syrinx was still distended and so a further aspiration was carried out and even paler yellow fluid obtained (protein 3.3 g/litre). Following this the whole of the cervical cord collapsed. Within 48 hours of the operation there was marked improvement in strength and sensation and to our surprise the tendon reflexes returned in his arms.

However, 3 months later he again noticed deterioration in the strength and feeling of his arms and when readmitted in February 1978 all movements of the right arm were weak, although the left arm was normal.

A second operation was carried out on 9 February 1978. A thoracic laminectomy was carried out from T2 to T6 inclusively. On opening the dura, distended cord was noticed in the upper part of the exposure while towards the middle of the exposure the cord was substituted by a syrinx. There was no cord substance visible, this being replaced by a fluid bag with translucent walls adjacent to a patent subarachnoid space. Immediately caudal to this area was a scarred atrophic cord with a wide surrounding subarachnoid space, partially obliterated by scar tissue (Figure 29). The most cranial syrinx was aspirated. Clear, colourless fluid was obtained this time with a protein content of 1.26 g/litre and 1.0 g/litre. Fluid from the surrounding subarachnoid space contained 2.3 g/litre of protein. The tough scarred area of cord containing the translucent membrane was excised and to our surprise a caudally directed syrinx was found. A soft polythene tube passed 6 cm down this syrinx whereas the cranially directed syrinx was 12 cm in length. There was noticeable improvement in strength and sensation within

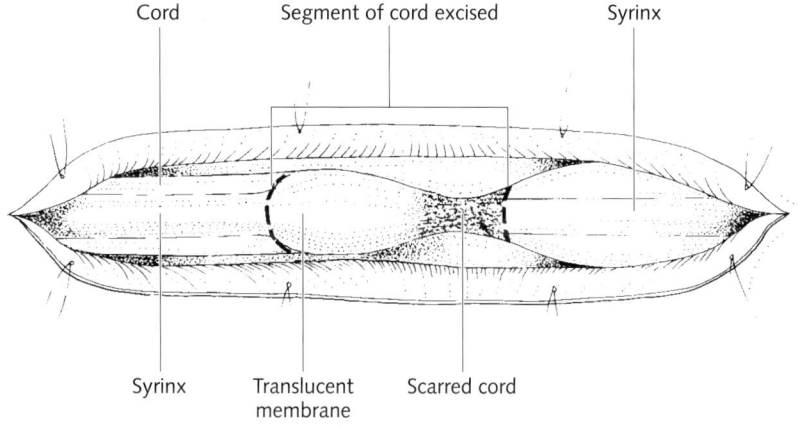

Cord   Segment of cord excised   Syrinx

Syrinx   Translucent membrane   Scarred cord

Fig. 29 Drawing to show the operative findings (see Figure 28).

48 hours and by 6 months post-operatively there were no abnormal signs in his arms.

This patient therefore had at least three cranially directed syrinxes and one caudally directed syrinx. They did not freely intercommunicate as shown by the differing protein contents and the failure of the cord to collapse by aspiration at just one site. It is of interest that at the first operation the syrinx fluid was yellow and of high protein content whereas at the second operation, 5 months later, it was clear and colourless and of a lower protein content. Excision of a damaged segment of cord and adjacent translucent membrane produced a persistent neurological improvement.

Translucent membranes

In these examples, both cranial and spinal, I have invariably found the cyst to be separated from the CSF by a translucent membrane. In the patient with a traumatic syrinx, the initial fluid was yellow but the subsequent fluid was clear and colourless, similar to CSF. One can envisage that initially an area of liquifactive necrosis of the brain or spinal cord forms and this may attract CSF by osmotic pressure across a translucent membrane. This of course requires the adjacent subarachnoid space to be patent and this may occur infrequently, thus providing an explanation for the relative rarity of these conditions. However, what mechanism allows these cysts to expand when the cyst contains clear, colourless fluid with a protein level identical to the CSF? These cysts expand sufficiently to displace intracranial structures, to cause raised intracranial pressure and to expand the overlying bone by remodelling. I do not know the answer but it seems to me that some active transport mechanism must exist across the translucent membrane.

Clearly more work needs to be done on this problem, but I mention these conditions to stimulate further thought amongst the next generation of neurosurgeons.

The cervical spine and spinal cord: movement and tethering

I have long been fascinated by the cervical spine. What a lot we do not know, and the number of worthwhile papers published on it have been so few. We need to know so much more about the basic mechanisms of cervical spondylotic radiculopathy and myelopathy. I resist the temptation to write about what is recorded in textbooks but will confine these notes to the normal dynamics of the spine, as well as the effects of tethering of the cervical dura and the influences that these factors have on the pathogenesis and treatment of cervical spondylotic radiculopathy and cervical spondylotic myelopathy.

Biomechanics of the cervical spine

The fact that the cervical spine is a most mobile structure is seemingly forgotten in many textbooks, especially pathological ones. The normal cervical spine moves up to 110° from extension into flexion and the head movement on the neck adds a further 30° on top of that. This is amazing! If one measures the posterior contour of the spinal canal between flexion and extension it expands by 5 cm while the anterior contour increases by 1.5 cm. Have you thought what happens to the cervical spinal cord and nerve roots to accommodate such changes?

Figure 30 explains what happens. In extension the dura is folded (and the cord is thicker) while in flexion the dura becomes taut and the cord thinner. In this way the dura and cord work like an accordion expanding and contracting. There is a further mechanism and that is that the cord and dural tube are pulled out of the thoracic spine during flexion. I am sure you have spoken to patients who describe exacerbation of their sciatica during flexion of the neck. The explanation is that the patient is pulling the cord and

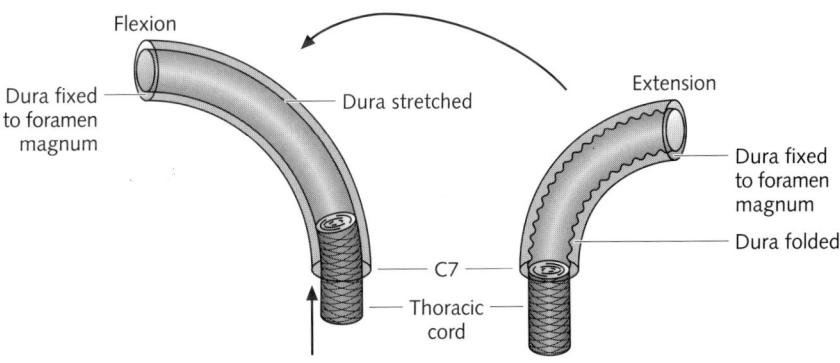

(1) Dural tube and cord unfold
(2) Dural tube and cord move from thoracic canal into cervical canal

Fig. 30 Diagram to show the biomechanical changes of the cervical cord and dura between extension and flexion. The dural tube (and cord) moves in and out like an accordion but also moves out of the thoracic spinal canal into the cervical spinal canal during flexion. It is firmly adherent at the foramen magnum.

thereby the lumbar nerve roots during cervical spine flexion. The dura is attached at the foramen magnum and also attached to the arachnoid, which makes dural decompression so difficult to achieve without penetrating the arachnoid, during a posterior fossa decompression for Arnold–Chiari malformation. The cord and dural tube move together at all times except at the foramen magnum where, during flexion the brain stem moves relatively to the dura into the spinal canal. Thus, neck flexion has been suggested as a test for incipient coning! I don't recommend it.

The intervertebral foramen

It is important to know that the intervertebral foramen, more accurately described as a canal as it is 1 cm in length, changes in size during movement of the neck. The cross-sectional area of the foramen becomes smaller during extension and the nerve root becomes thicker. Hence, the characteristic feature of cervical radiculopathy is that the pain and pins and needles down the arm are brought on with extension of the neck, for instance, during shaving under the chin.

Another useful fact is that the foramen between congenitally fused vertebrae is extremely small and the patient never develops a radiculopathy at that level. This has important therapeutic implications in so much that it is not necessary for the surgeon to increase the foraminal size by drilling away osteophytes, to stop radiculopathy pain. All that is necessary is to create a fusion which is a much safer operation than a procedure that entails drilling away osteophytes adjacent to the spinal cord.

I find it useful to carry out lateral cervical spine radiographs in full flexion and extension. By superimposing these two radiographs one can quickly and accurately assess the biomechanics of a cervical spine (Figure 31). It is remarkable how often surgeons consider an anterior cervical fusion without knowing if the joint in question is mobile or not!

Tethered cervical cord syndrome

As a young man I was interested in a group of patients with cervical spondylotic myelopathy who deteriorated neurologically about 2 years after decompressive laminectomy. Comparing the group of patients who derived dramatic and sustained benefit from the laminectomy and those who showed delayed neurological deterioration, it was apparent that the latter group either had the dura opened or the range of movement of the head and neck in the sagittal plane was over 40°. I suggested that decompressive laminectomy

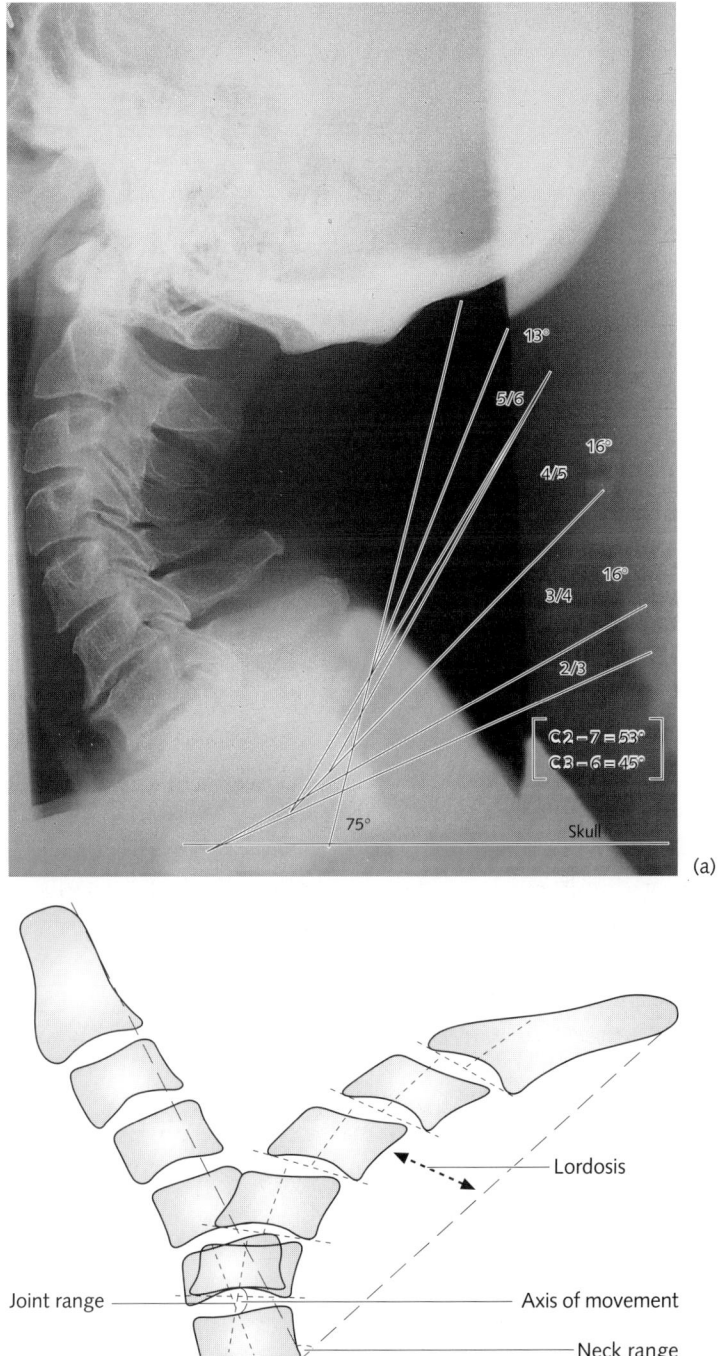

Labels within figure (a):
13°
5/6
16°
4/5
16°
3/4
2/3
C2−7 = 53°
C3−6 = 45°
75°
Skull

(a)

Labels within figure (b):
Lordosis
Joint range
Axis of movement
Neck range

Additional information obtained from flexion–extension radiographs (b)

Fig. 31 (a,b) Measurements can be quickly and accurately made from lateral flexion and extension radiographs of the cervical spine. One radiograph is superimposed on the other at C7 vertebrae: a line is drawn along the back of the margin of the upper radiograph onto the lower radiograph. The radiographs are then superimposed at C6 and a further line drawn, etc.

performed on a mobile cervical spine was likely to eventually cause a traction injury to the cord and hence neurological deterioration. The mechanism of this, I believe, is adherence of the cervical dura to the muscle, or if the dura is opened, the cord itself to the muscle (Figure 32). The dura is fixed at the foramen magnum and when a high range of movement is regained once the post-operative pain and stiffness have receded, traction damage occurs to the tethered cord during flexion.

This 'tethered cervical cord syndrome' produces a collection of symptoms and signs due to a mixture of upper and lower motor neurone features. I have seen this syndrome after cervical laminectomy for not only spondylotic myelopathy but laminectomy for tumours. It is extremely difficult to treat; I have eventually resorted to multiple anterior cervical fusions to reduce the range of movement of the spine. As far as I know this syndrome is not described in any textbook. I suspect it is under-diagnosed but by describing it here I hope it will be recognized more in the future.

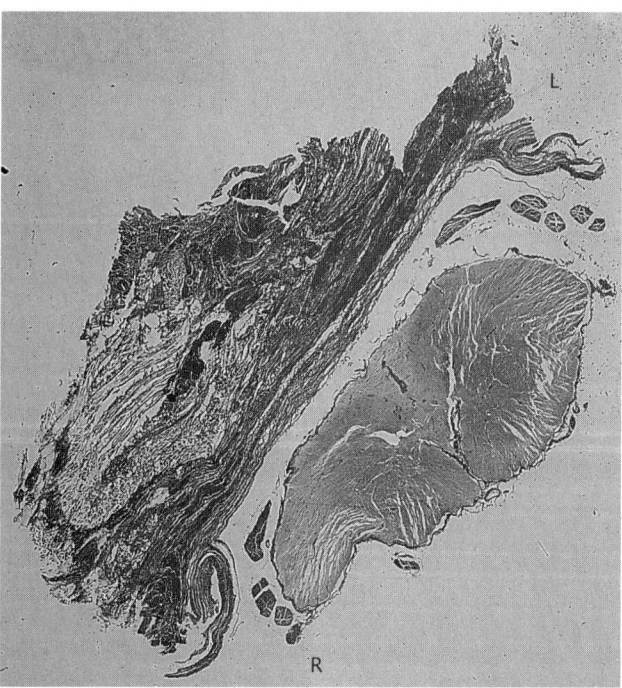

Fig. 32 Post-mortem photograph to show the adherence of the dura to the muscle following a cervical laminectomy. This destroys the normal physiological movement of the dura.

Cervical spondylotic myelopathy

We have a poor understanding of the pathogenesis of this common condition. One factor that I believe to be of the greatest importance is movement. I stress this factor as it has been consistently ignored by the majority of surgeons. The MRI scan has for the first time, given us a test to confirm the diagnosis of spondylotic myelopathy by demonstrating spinal cord damage opposite a disc space. The clinical picture is usually characteristic with the onset of paraesthesia in the fingers, lack of facility of movement of the hands and stiffness of the legs. The mechanism of the glove and stocking loss, characteristic of this condition (as well as peripheral neuropathy), has never been fully explained.

Clearly, the narrowing of the canal by osteophytes is also an important factor but this is not enough. Osteophytes and movement are important. Usually cord damage occurs in extension, but there is a group where cord damage seems to occur in flexion (Figure 33). Of course there is a further group of patients where the myelopathy occurs because of an unstable subluxation, and a fusion at this level produces an excellent result.

If the mechanism is essentially compression due to a narrow canal then one would expect a decompressive laminectomy to be extremely successful. In general it is not a satisfactory procedure except in the group of patients with a diffusely narrow cervical canal that is relatively immobile. This is a rather small group because we know that relative immobility is a protection against neurological deterioration. Furthermore, as I have mentioned, decompressive laminectomy in the presence of a mobile spine may in fact produce neurological damage itself due to traction of the tethered cord.

I believe the correct procedure should be designed for each patient on the basis of the biomechanical factors operating for that particular patient (Table 8). I gave a lecture once at a prestigious department of neurosurgery in North America. My view that movement was an important factor in the pathogenesis of cervical spondylotic myelopathy clearly did not impress the surgeons who said that they had excellent results from doing a decompressive laminectomy. After the lecture the Professor of Neurology came round to thank me for the lecture, saying that the results of surgery for cervical spondylotic myelopathy were so bad that he had stopped referring patients for surgery! This is an example of selection, for clearly the surgeons were getting excellent results in that subgroup of patients with a diffusely narrow, relatively immobile spinal canal but were not seeing many other patients with this condition.

I often tell patients that it may be necessary to do a two-stage procedure.

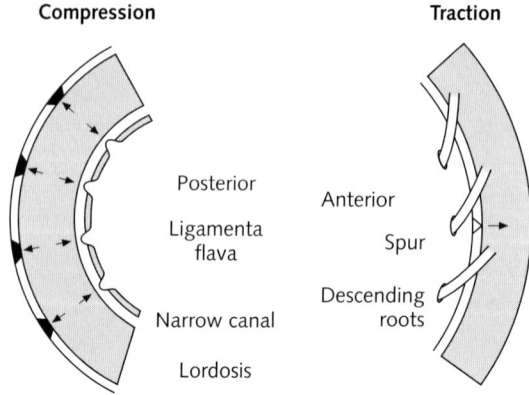

Compression   Traction

Posterior

Ligamenta
flava

Narrow canal

Lordosis

Anterior

Spur

Descending
roots

MYELOPATHY

1. Compression in extension
1. Narrow spinal canal
2. High range of movement – into extension
3. Marked lordosis in extension

2. Traction in flexion
1. Osteophyte at summit of kyphosis
2. Descending extrathecal nerve roots i.e. tense cord
3. High range of movement of the head and neck into flexion, *or*
4. marked kyphosis in flexion

Fig. 33 Pathogenesis of cervical spondylotic myelopathy, usually during extension but occasionally it may occur during flexion.

Table 8 The appropriate treatment of cervical spondylotic myelopathy depending on the biomechanics: laminoplasty is probably better than a decompressive laminectomy because it reduces adherence of the dura to the muscle and is also a safer option.

Subluxation—fusion

Damage in extension
High range of movement
    Fusion of most mobile, relevant, intervertebral joints
    Later, if necessary, decompressive laminectomy/laminoplasty

Low range of movement
    Conservative approach; less likely to progress
    Decompressive laminectomy/laminoplasty

Damage in flexion
Collar
Fusion of most mobile intervertebral joints

The first stage is a one- or two- (occasionally three) level anterior fusion and if that is unsuccessful then a decompression would be done at a second stage when the range of movement of the spine has been reduced by the fusion and the 'tethered dura/cord' complications would be less likely to occur. These days I prefer a suspension laminoplasty because I believe there is less dural adhesion to the muscle following this procedure and there seems to be a much better restoration of the subarachnoid space posterior to the cervical spinal cord following this procedure compared with a decompressive laminectomy. It is also a safer procedure; at least in my hands there is a lower incidence of spinal cord damage compared with a decompressive laminectomy.

Cusick *et al.* produced a momentous paper; they took patients bedridden with cervical spondylotic myelopathy and fused their heads and necks without any attempt to decompress the spinal cord. The patients all became ambulatory, which demonstrates the importance of movement of the head and neck in the pathogenesis and treatment of this condition.

I do not think papers comparing anterior fusion with decompressive laminectomy are useful. We need more papers analysing the biomechanical factors and the best way of treating these. It would be instructive to take two groups of patients, one group comprising patients who had dramatically improved and compare the biomechanics with a group of patients who had failed to show improvement. This type of study, I believe, will provide much worthwhile information.

Cervical spondylotic radiculopathy

The results of surgery for cervical spondylotic radiculopathy are much more satisfactory than for myelopathy. I personally find anterior discectomy and fusion to be remarkably effective. I use a bone graft from the patient's iliac crest and make no effort to remove osteophytes, but I always look for extruded disc fragments by incising the posterior longitudinal ligament and gently probing with a blunt hook. Although I do attempt to increase the cross-sectional area of the foramen by maintaining the width of the distract-ed disc space by using a suitably shaped bone graft, I am not sure I am always successful in achieving this aim, nor am I sure that it is particularly important to achieve this. Almost certainly, the cessation of movement is much more important than the increase in foraminal cross-sectional area.

One final comment before leaving cervical radiculopathy; the MRI scan does not always give a clear picture of the pathology and indeed the MRI changes may be diffuse but only pathological at one level. You must not rely on the MRI scan but on the history and examination! Chapter 3 dwells on the history and examination because it is so important, and I frequently advise surgery on the basis of the history and examination (especially using the reflex changes, which are, in general, so reliable) if the MRI scan is unclear. I have never regretted this approach. Occasionally I do this as well when dealing with sciatica. Thank goodness the MRI scan is not always diagnostic. It makes life much more challenging and interesting!

However, occasionally the clinical features can mislead. A patient, a doctor, had a clear C7 root lesion clinically. The MRI scan showed a para-central disc prolapse at C5/6, which would normally affect the C6 root. However, the clinical features in this patient were, I believe, due to damage of the C7 rootlets intrathecally rather than in the intervertebral canal, hence the misleading level on clinical assessment; the C7 rootlets intrathecally are at the C5/6 level rather than lower down. Beware of this then, with paracentral disc prolapses compared with more lateral disc prolapses!

Lumbar disc prolapse

You would be forgiven for being surprised that there is anything that could be written in this section that is not already well described in textbooks and in everyday use in this, the most common, neurosurgical condition. There are three aspects, however, that I believe are not commonly known or used which I have found of immense help. The first I have already mentioned and that is how to test for power of dorsiflexion of the foot. Most neurologists and neurosurgeons do not know how to do this. 'So what?', I hear you say, 'With MRI scans you don't need to worry about this'. That is just the point; the more sophisticated the tests the more important it is to treat the patient and not the scan, and the only way to treat the patient is to take a history and examine the patient.

There is one important, practical tip to mention. If you operate on a patient with an L4/5 disc prolapse and do not find a disc prolapse, go down to the 'L5/S1' level, and you will find it there. This worrying scenario occurs when L5 is fused (congenitally) to the sacrum so the last mobile joint is in fact the L4/5 level and not L5/S1. This fusion may not be obvious on the scan but a clue is a very normal-looking L5/S1 disc (not dehydrated) on the MRI scan. This suggests no movement is occurring at this level. Congenital fusion of L5 to S1 is a source of considerable confusion! I have seen patients operated on by senior, experienced neurosurgeons who have failed to find the relevant disc prolapse because they have not realized L5 was fused to the sacrum and they were in fact exploring the L3/4 disc space instead of the L4/5 space.

Most people think lumbar disc surgery is easy; I don't. It may be easy but it may be hard. A lot of operating depends on 'feel': what feels normal and what does not; also how tissues feel and how much manipulation of tissues is safe. Lumbar spine surgery is more difficult than doing a craniotomy when you start operating because a lot of the operation is knowing the normal feel and you do not know this until you have done a reasonable number! Also feel gently. Do not run a dissector along the extradural space or you will rupture those epidural veins. Instead feel by bringing the dissector in and out. When removing disc material press the rongeurs against the vertebral body; I am sure you know why you should not push the ronguers too far anteriorly!

I prefer a decent exposure when carrying out lumbar disc surgery for two reasons. First, it reduces the risk of missing a disc fragment and allows a more complete removal of disc material, but perhaps of more importance, it allows a good decompression of the nerve root, which allows safer retraction as well as better post-operative relief of pain. I never mind removing the medial half of a facet joint on one side to obtain adequate decompression and please do not remove a central disc prolapse through a fenestration. I have seen too many patients develop a post-operative cauda equina syndrome because of an inadequate bony decompression. I always carry out a full laminectomy in these circumstances.

Curable back pain

The art of taking a history leads me to the second point. It is well known that good, indeed excellent, results occur when the surgeon finds and removes a chunk of extruded disc compressing the nerve root. The leg pain goes immediately. Indeed we do back operations for leg pain, not back pain and in lumbar disc surgery the emphasis should be on finding those patients with nerve root compression: if the symptoms (sciatica, pins and needles) and physical signs (L5 or S1 usually) fit with the MRI scan appearance then there is a 99% chance of the patient's sciatica being relieved by operation. It is best to wait 6 weeks before advising operation because the symptoms may well resolve in this time but if they have not, then without surgery they tend to drag on. Generally back operations for back pain, and this usually means fusion procedures for lumbar spondylosis, are very disappointing in terms of relief of pain. However, there is a group of patients with curable back pain due to a central disc prolapse. When one takes a careful history from a patient with sciatica (i.e. pain that extends below the knee) one often obtains a history, often for years, of episodic back pain which then culminates in sciatica and often at that point the back pain improves or goes. I consider the back pain is caused by the annulus fibrosus rupturing allowing the nucleus pulposus to distort the pain-sensitive posterior longitudinal ligament. Further protrusion of the disc distorts the nerve root causing sciatica.

There is a group of patients with centrally placed disc prolapses who only suffer back pain and because of this they are often not investigated and consequently denied a cure. There are two characteristic features that allow a high degree of clinical certainty of a central disc prolapse. These are: first, the patient can remember precisely the initial event, so that prior to the event there was no back pain and subsequent to the event, episodic back pain. Secondly, the back pain is characterized by being worse on sitting. Driving a car for any length of time becomes impossible.

Investigations show a well-marked, clear-cut, central disc prolapse, usually at the L4/5 interspace. Removal of this usually cures the back pain.

The first patient I had was a doctor, who as a medical student had lifted a heavy object and since then had increasingly severe episodes of back pain. Twenty years later he was finding he could no longer sit to do his surgeries. A myelogram showed a large central disc prolapse; 6 weeks after its removal he was playing tennis, something he had been unable to do for several years. Another case was a woman who clearly remembered that her back pain started 29 years previously whilst changing a nappy on her baby. An MRI scan confirmed the central disc prolapse and she obtained instant relief from removal of the prolapse. A third example is the man who 17 years previously had a hot shower, then bent down to put his (then) young daughter on the potty. As he did so he bent forward and slightly turned. At that moment his back 'went'. 'Pre-potty', no back pain; 'post-potty', episodes of back pain culminating in a severe episode so that he was off work because he could not sit down. The MRI scan (Figure 34) showed a central disc prolapse, removal of which cured the back pain. These patients are not numerous but are, I believe, not being diagnosed, which denies them relief of their curable back pain.

Making laminectomy pain free

Why not make operations on the lumbar spine pain free? Most patients will confess to fairly unpleasant back pain following operations on the lumbar spine. My personal preference is to do a laminectomy for a disc prolapse in preference to a microdiscectomy, as, I believe, the relief of pain is better

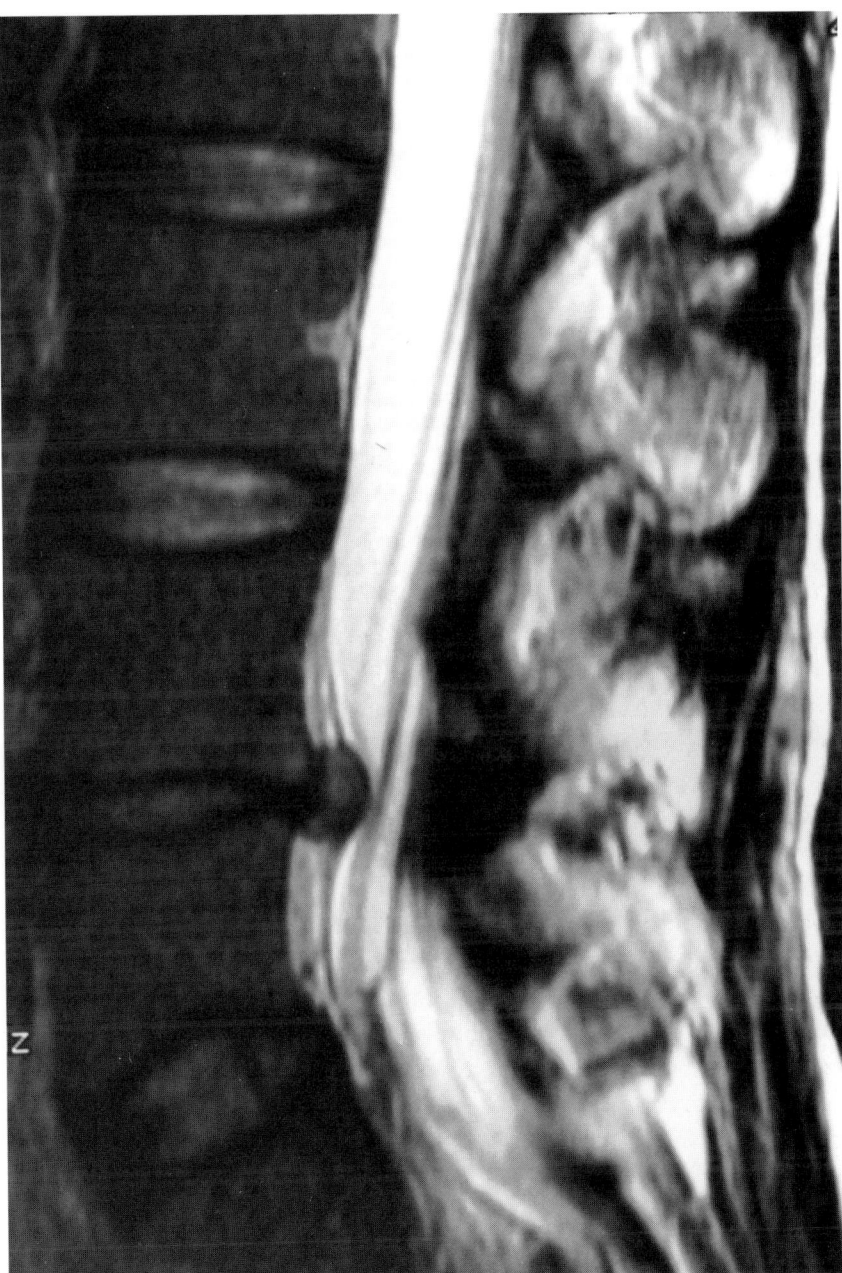

Fig. 34 Central disc prolapse causing just back pain. This occurred 17 years before the operation when the patient bent forward and twisted to place his daughter on the potty.

(because a good decompression of the nerve root can be achieved), the risk of nerve damage is less (for the same reason) and the recurrence rate is lower because a better clearance of the adjacent disc material can be obtained. But irrespective of which technique is used, and of course decompressive laminectomies are necessary for conditions such as spinal stenosis, back operations are painful and the problem with 'patient-controlled analgesia' is that when the patient goes to sleep they wake up in pain. Pain relief is important not just for moral and humanitarian reasons but also because it allows the patient to mobilize quickly, minimizing stiffness and this in itself reduces back pain.

For a number of years I have been inserting epidural catheters at the time of surgery and then giving post-operative diamorphine. Initially this was given as a bolus every 8 hours but the use of the 'epifuser' has made the technique easier and more effective (Figure 35). The infusion lasts for 3 days and removes most, if not all, post-operative pain. It allows the patient to get up the following day and many patients tell me that the last pain they had was the anaesthetist's needle at the time of induction of anaesthesia. At the time of the operation, the epidural catheter (Baxter, John Radcliffe epidural set) is inserted in a cranial direction so that the '4 line' marker is at the level of the skin, the catheter being inserted through a separate stab incision. The catheter is then flushed with saline to ensure patency and to ensure that saline is not seen to emerge in the wound where it would be removed by the suction drain. The technique involves a 2-mg diamorphine bolus (in 5 ml saline) injection down the epidural catheter with the suction drain switched off for 20 minutes. This is given in the recovery room. Twenty milligrams of diamorphine in 250 ml of 5% dextrose saline is placed into the 'epifuser', which then supplies a small dose of diamorphine over the following 3 days. Care must be taken to watch the respiratory rate, although with this regimen we have had to give naloxone only very occasionally. Sometimes patients 'itch' from the diamorphine but are usually prepared to accept an itch for pain relief. Occasionally male patients develop retention of urine; they do so anyway after back operations at times and the incidence of this can be reduced by restricting the amount of fluids given at operation. I am not convinced that the incidence of retention is higher using epidural analgesia but a urinary catheter for 3 days is worth it for the superb relief of pain. I avoid using this technique if the dura has been opened. Initially we were very circumspect in using this technique for patients over the age of 65 years but with increasing experience we are now much less concerned, although we reduce the dose in those over 65 years of age to a 1- or 1.5-mg bolus and 15 mg into the epifuser (Table 9).

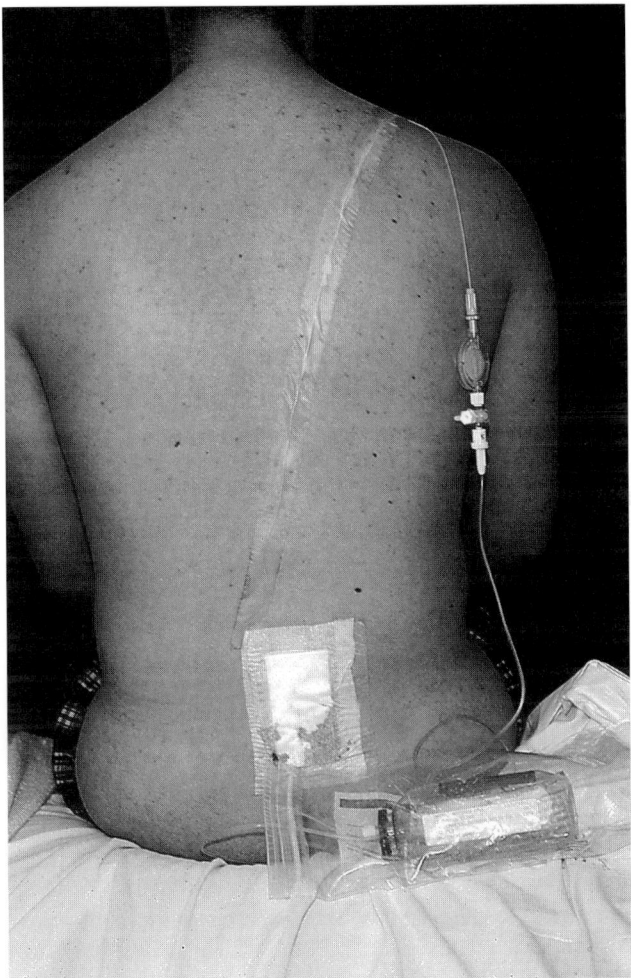

Fig. 35 Pain-free lumbar laminectomy! The 'epifuser' injects a continuous supply of diamorphine into the epidural space for 3 days, which allows the patient to mobilize without any pain.

Pain-free cervical laminectomy

I have also started to use epidural analgesia after cervical laminectomy or laminoplasty (Figure 36). I insert the epidural catheter caudally and use the same diamorphine regimen. Why this should work in these circumstances, being passed caudally, I do not know, but it does. It raises interesting questions as to the mechanism of pain relief. The advantage of this technique is that it is extremely effective, provides the analgesia where it is needed rather

Table 9 Epidural diamorphine infusion: how to deal with complications.

All epidural infusions should have a three-way tap distal to the epidural filter so that the infusion can be turned off and on. A regular back-up non-steroidal anti-inflammatory drug (NSAID) means that the patient needs less opioid and that when the infusion wears off, he or she is not left without analgesia. (Courtesy of Jean Millar, Consultant Anaesthetist.)

Problem	Remedy
Respiration <8/minute	• Turn off epidural • Give naloxone 0.2 mg if the patient does not respond to commands to breathe
Patient still has mild pain	• Give oral analgesics such as co-proxamol • Make sure the patient is receiving a regular NSAID (i.e. diclofenac)
The pain does not respond to these, or the pain is severe	• Turn off the wound suction drain • Consider giving another 1–2 mg diamorphine epidurally • If these are unsuccessful, change to patient-controlled analgesia
Nausea	• Give ondansetron or cyclizine, or both if necessary • If the nausea continues and the patient is not in pain, turn off the epidural for 1–2 hours
Itch	• If the patient is not in pain turn off the epidural for 1–2 hours • 0.1 mg naloxone IV if severe • Piriton may help
The patient has not passed urine, but is comfortable	• Do not worry in the first 24 hours • Mobilize the patient and allow him or her to go to the lavatory—this usually works if you (and the patient) are patient • If it does not, turn off the epidural for 1–2 hours
The patient cannot pass urine despite these measures *and* is uncomfortable	• Catheterize • Continue with epidural

than flooding the whole patient with opiates and is extremely safe because the diamorphine is inserted into the epifuser by the anaesthetist at the time of the operation and does not require any further introduction of diamorphine. Try it—your patients will thank you!

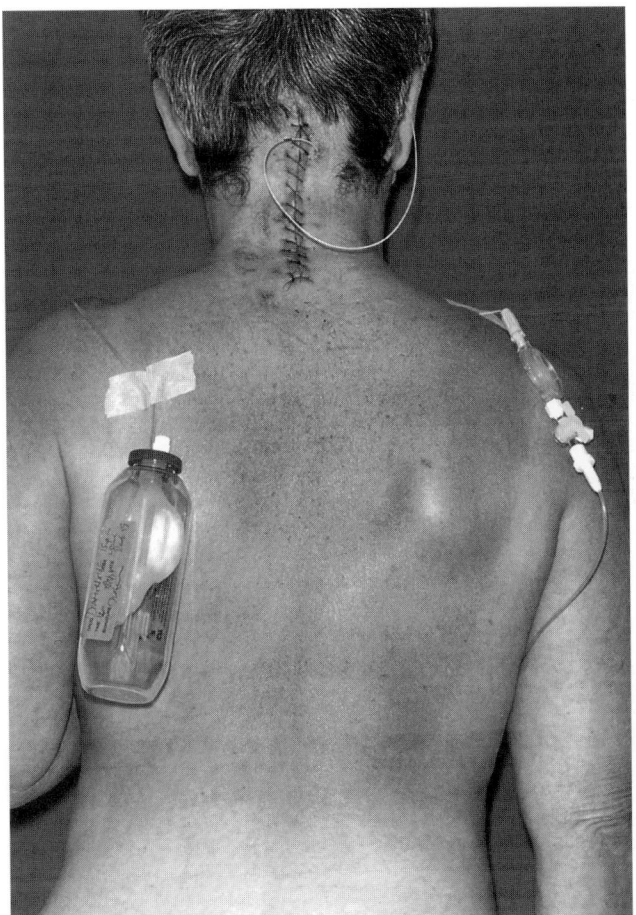

Fig. 36 This technique can also be used after cervical laminectomy or laminoplasty. The patient had her operation the previous day. The epidural catheter is passed caudally to the mid-thoracic region. The fact it works so well raises interesting questions as to how it works. This is usually a particularly painful operation.

Spinal arteriovenous malformations

In the old, myelogram, days, the dye was (or should have been) taken to the mid-thoracic region to exclude this condition. I worry that MRI scans for sciatica, confined to the lumbar region, will miss these curable lesions. Always think of this if you have a patient with a story of cauda equina claudication (pain on standing or walking relieved by sitting or lying) without spinal stenosis being found. The acquired form of spinal arteriovenous malformation occurs in the same age group. The fistula is extradural (Figure 37) and the patients do well from operation, which is very safe and straightforward.

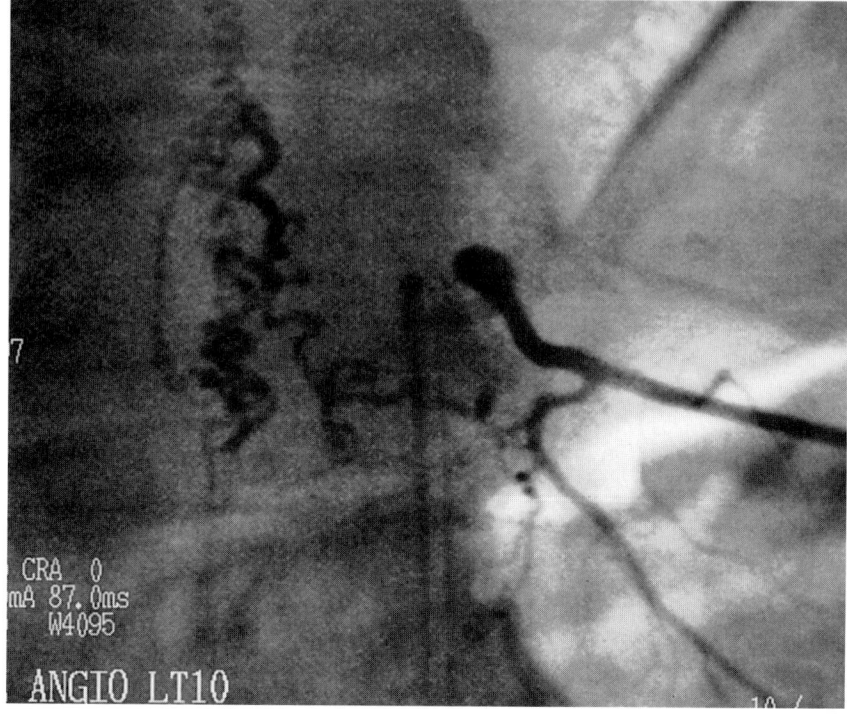

Fig. 37 Spinal angiogram to show an 'acquired' spinal AVM due to an extradural fistula with the draining vein reaching the spinal cord along the nerve root. These may present as 'cauda equina claudication without spinal stenosis'.

The operation entails finding the draining vein on the nerve root and tracing this back to the dura. The fistula, extradurally sited, can be excised and a short segment of the intradural draining vein excised. The spinal cord does not need to be touched.

A few maverick spinal thoughts

Lumbar fusion

Lumbar fusion for back pain due to lumbar spondylosis is a miserably disappointing procedure. I avoid it like the plague as only 50% of patients are helped. Instead of thinking up new and more expensive forms of scaffolding, surgeons would be far better off trying to work out the mechanism of spondylotic back pain and how to choose those patients who will be helped. Even more important is to realize (and tell the patients!) that this back pain is episodic and that it will, in fact, get better as they get older. This is true for the cervical spine as well as the lumbar spine. In fact the worse the MRI scan appearance the less the pain because the spondylosis has produced a natural fusion (or at least stiffening), which seems far better at stopping pain than a surgical fusion: another excellent reason for not operating on the scan but on patients! Very often patients feel that if they have this amount of low back pain now, then surely they will be much worse in 5 or 10 years' time. Tell the patients that, in fact, they will be better in 5 or 10 years' time, not worse (very often this is all they need to know), that they will not be in a wheelchair (it never ceases to amaze me that patients are told this wicked lie by surgeons) and that by taking exercise they will be helping, not harming, themselves even though they may get some pain during activity.

Down's syndrome

It is important to know that occasionally these people may be unstable at C1–C2, and may develop symptoms and signs of cord compression at this level. Do not do a laminectomy, but do a fusion. I do not think they need a trans-oral removal of their odontoid peg either. Dare I say it, but I think this operation is rather over-done and patients who undergo this operation (for any reason other than tumour) often need a good fusion (from behind) rather than both a fusion and removal of the odontoid peg.

Tethered cord, adhesions and fat grafts

Before I leave the spine I have two more sceptical confessions to make. First, I have grave reservations about 'tethered cords' in spina bifida occulta and the need to release them. I need facts to convince me, not emotion please! Secondly, epidural adhesions after lumbar disc surgery do not cause post-operative pain! Every patient, even those who are entirely pain free, get epidural adhesions—if you don't believe me look at a few post-operative MRI scans. So do not waste time putting in fat grafts. Intradural (and intraneural) scarring does cause pain. Rough surgery produces this scarring so be gentle with nerve roots, and do a good decompression before retracting them! Arachnoiditis (or intradural scarring) is a miserable condition and is untreatable.

The cause of post-operative continuation of pre-operative pain is poor selection and is your (or my) fault! If a patient has symptoms and signs of nerve root compression that fit with the MRI scan appearance, then they have a 98% chance of losing their sciatica.

Neurofibromatosis

I make just one comment: think not once, but at least three times before doing laminectomy to remove one of the numerous spinal tumours. Usually these tumours do not need removing. These patients' spines are potentially unstable and a laminectomy may be disastrous. Signs of cord damage may be due to the kyphoscoliosis these patients develop and not the tumours. Again, never operate on scans but on patients!

chapter nine

Operative hints and suggestions

General hints and suggestions

The KISS principle ('keep it simple and safe') is important when deciding which operation to perform. It is also important during the operation. Simplicity means safety. It also means that the surgeon has a clear understanding of what can or cannot be achieved. Neurosurgery also requires that the surgeon avoid difficulties if at all possible as well as knowing how to deal with the difficulties if they occur. It is much easier to avoid problems. These can be best avoided before the surgeon picks up the knife, by careful pre-operative assessment, the correct choice of operation as well as the correct siting of the incision.

Plan the incision and the position of the patient

Failure to place the incision correctly can make life extremely difficult and convert a straightforward operation into a lengthy and tedious one. The surgeon is well advised to plan the incision and position the patient himself. I find the sitting or reclining position helpful to reduce the venous pressure but one is always worried about air embolism.

Avoiding air embolism

I personally use the sitting position and have done so for 25 years without significant air embolism. I choose my cases and my anaesthetist. I only use the sitting position for strictly midline exposures. My anaesthetists are experienced. Doppler monitoring and end tidal CO_2 recording as well as a central line are used. The prevention of air embolism depends on an experienced surgeon as well as an experienced anaesthetist. For instance if I see an open vein I quickly occlude it and ask the anaesthetist to squeeze the neck in order to elevate the venous pressure. If there is little bleeding then I am especially vigilant and warn the anaesthetist of the potential danger of air embolism. The operating conditions are so good that the extra trouble taken to avoid an air embolism is in my view well worthwhile. The sitting position is especially useful for the supracerebellar subtentorial approach to pineal tumours, the procedure of choice in my opinion for such lesions. The reclining position with the patient pinned from behind is useful as well. I like to keep the head straight (rather than twisting it) whenever I can because I can appreciate the anatomical relationships more easily this way.

A good surgeon

Surgery should never be hurried, but the sign of a good surgeon is one who does an unhurried operation quickly. This is achieved by economy of movement, avoiding difficulties, knowing what needs doing, doing it and then closing up! There is no doubt that an operation done quickly is better for the patient, with less chance of infection as long as it is not hurried. Surgeons when they start, tend to make many cuts rather than one. Many scalpel cuts take longer and cause more tissue damage and bleeding. Aim to make just one cut whenever possible!

Do you give antibiotics?

I now give all my patients prophylactic antibiotics. For operations traversing air sinuses I give a 5-day course. For most operations the patient receives a single dose of antibiotics during the induction of anaesthesia. This has virtually irradicated that most unpleasant condition of 'discitis', which used to occur after lumbar disc removal. Discitis, a low-grade infection of a disc space, causes severe back 'spasms' (no sciatica and quite unlike any preoperative pain) usually 1 or 2 weeks after the operation. Resolution slowly occurs and leads to a bony fusion across the disc space, which is the only time this occurs spontaneously in my experience. When this happens the patient becomes entirely pain free.

To stage or not to stage?

Sometimes staging operations can make things easier for the surgeon and safer for the patient. Everyone, I believe, would agree endovascular treatment (one or more times) is helpful prior to the definitive operation for a large intracerebral arteriovenous malformation (AVM). But should one stage operations? In general I think not but there are exceptions. For instance a suprasellar meningioma wrapped around both internal carotid arteries and its branches is better staged, first one side, then the other. An anteriorly placed foramen magnum meningioma approached postero-laterally along the line of each vertebral artery is probably better staged, first one side, then the other. Equally, some pituitary tumours may be staged; a trans-sphenoidal approach followed by a trans-cranial. All these examples of staging are imposed by the anatomical situation and extent of the tumour rather than the pathology. Once I am involved with accessible pathology, I am reluctant to stop unless other factors are relevant.

These other factors are, for instance, blood loss and disturbance of function. Once, I had a 9-year-old girl with a massive falcine and parasagittal meningioma presenting with such a large swelling of the vertex of the skull that her hair was piled up over it to disguise it. I removed this tumour in three stages: the first to remove the involved bone (which involved a large blood loss), the second to remove the left-sided tumour and the third to remove the remaining tumour and involved sagittal sinus. Very often it pays to remove a large bilateral parasagittal meningioma in stages, first to prevent possible post-operative paraplegia and secondly to allow the venous circulation to re-establish itself after the first operation. Of course if part of the posterior two-thirds of the superior sagittal sinus is patent yet involved with tumour, then it is often better to carry out a subtotal removal and wait for the recurrence to slowly block the sinus before attempting a total removal.

On the other hand I would not stage the removal of an acoustic neuroma, however large or vascular it was. In these circumstances the obliteration of the normal tissue planes around the tumour by the first operation would make a second stage much more difficult. It is well known, and a true adage, that the best chance of removing a tumour is the first operation, unless of course other factors mentioned above are relevant. In summary, there are no fixed rules and surgical judgement is needed for each patient.

Basic technique

I have a very standardized technique for turning a bone flap. After each layer I stop the bleeding. It is a remarkable example of DNA coding how every patient seems to have the same tiny vessels in the same place and one soon learns where to look for them. Once the dura is opened I place a layer of Surgicel over the brain. This allows inexpensive patties to be used to protect the brain and the Surgicel allows the patties to be removed easily and atraumatically from the brain surface. There are more expensive patties available which are very nice to use but my method is cheaper and just as effective!

Retractors

Self-retaining retractors are essential but there are dangers in their use. One must always remember the capillary circulation under the retractor blade is what counts. A retractor should never be placed directly on the brain. Avoid using two retractors if at all possible and especially during aneurysm surgery. There is an increased chance of rupturing the aneurysm if two retractors are used pulling in different directions. Never have a retractor in unless it is necessary. For instance when operating on the fifth nerve in the posterior fossa, I do not use a retractor and rely on sucking away the cerebrospinal fluid (CSF) whilst gently retracting the cerebellum using a sucker applied to a patty resting on a Surgicel-covered surface of the cerebellum.

The operating microscope

The operating microscope has of course transformed neurosurgery. As a young surgeon and an enthusiastic microneurosurgeon, I was warned by one of my chiefs that the operating microscope would make operations even longer with a greater infection rate. The converse is true; the operations are shorter, incomparably less traumatic and allow us to achieve so much more. I learned never to reject an advance out of hand after that!

Suction

Like most surgeons using the operating microscope I use a sucker in my left hand and either bipolar forceps or microscissors in my right hand. I like the sucker to be electrically controlled so that I can obtain effective suction with the least trauma to the tissues. I tend to use the sucker as a retractor, especially when splitting the Sylvian fissure. On other occasions such as debulking a malignant glioma I find a 'two-sucker technique' useful. I have a more powerful sucker in my right hand with the unipolar diathermy applied to it. This allows the tumour to be debulked and to coagulate the pathological vessels by using the side of the end of the sucker, the field being kept dry with the left hand sucker. Using a sucker with the unipolar diathermy applied is extremely useful when carrying out a cortical resection or indeed when dealing with epidural veins in the spine. I call this 'the poor man's laser' but there are probably more lasers gathering dust in neurosurgical theatres than any other surgical instrument.

Which instruments do you need?

I believe that any surgeon can perform world-class neurosurgery with a good microscope, a self-retaining retractor, microinstruments and bipolar coagulation. One does not need anything else. I have stopped using the ultrasonic aspirator and much prefer debulking a meningioma or acoustic neuroma with the bipolar coagulation, especially with built-in irrigation. I believe the sucker, when used properly is a wonderful instrument but all too frequently the assistant feels that he or she has to do something. 'Something' usually means wielding the sucker with the enthusiasm usually associated with stirring the Christmas pudding. It indeed becomes an addiction for some assistants and I usually have to forbid the use of the sucker in these circumstances for it often causes more bleeding and tissue damage.

Blood loss

The measurement of blood loss is difficult; I have never lost a patient from over-transfusion but I have lost two children from under-transfusion. These patients collapsed in the ward 3 or 4 hours after the surgery and after their passage through the recovery room. Adams' Law of (paediatric) Blood Loss is to ask the anaesthetist how much blood he or she thinks the patient has lost, and then double it. This comes out to be about the correct amount that the patient needs.

Finding and maintaining the correct plane

This is perhaps the key to removing benign tumours. The correct plane for a meningioma is in fact the subdural plane and you do not need (as many books say) to cut the arachnoid. You can confirm this for yourself when you remove a small meningioma that has not ulcerated through the arachnoid, pia and even the cortex. It is better to gently retract the tumour away from the brain rather than the reverse. In order to do this you may need to debulk the tumour but if the tumour is soft (i.e. a cavernous angioma) it is compressible, and debulking is not necessary. If you get into bleeding you have probably lost the correct plane and wandered into tumour or brain. Go somewhere else, find the correct plane and work yourself along to the previous place where you lost the plane. A constant question to ask is 'does this vessel belong to the tumour or the brain'?

Maintaining a plane of dissection requires three things: patience, gentleness and a bloodless field. Never hurry and never lose your cool! One great advantage of the operating microscope is that it allows the surgeon to creep to the origin of the (say a suprasellar meningioma) tumour and detach it from its origin, and its blood supply. Of course pre-operative embolization may help. Unfortunately this is not possible when dealing with a large vascular acoustic neuroma. These tumours obtain some of their blood supply from the dura around the internal auditory meatus (via the external and internal carotid arteries), and so detaching the tumour from the meatus may help. I have no hesitation in asking the anaesthetist to drop the blood pressure if I find the bleeding troublesome. Indeed this has been of immense benefit when dealing with a vascular acoustic neuroma. At the end of the operation ask the anaesthetist to bring the blood pressure up to over 100 systolic to check the bleeding. Remember hypotension, you will be pleased you did one day!

There is one occasion when attempting to find the plane may be impossible and indeed dangerous: this is removing a meningioma from the brain stem. Sometimes the tumour peels away easily. Other times it does not. My advice is, if it does not and the attempts result in the pia being damaged, then desist. It is preferable to leave a thin layer of tumour stuck on to the vessels and brain stem in these circumstances. I have regretted ignoring this advice in the past.

Stopping pathological bleeding

Many of the methods used to stop pathological bleeding have been mentioned elsewhere in this notebook. Perhaps it is convenient to summarize these. Pre-operative embolization of a tumour is helpful, if possible, but should be done no longer than 2 or 3 days before the operation, and the tumour usually needs an external carotid arterial supply. Cut off the blood supply of a meningioma as soon as possible. The operating microscope helps to do this: one suprasellar meningioma was supplied by a single artery arising from the internal carotid artery near the ophthalmic artery. Early coagulation of this vessel devascularized the whole tumour. 'Getting in the right plane' reduces bleeding when removing benign tumours and if you wander out of the right plane you are rewarded by bleeding. When removing a glioblastoma or a pituitary tumour, do not worry about the bleeding because it will stop once the tumour has been removed! Do not try and stop the bleeding as you go, be bold and continue to remove the tumour and the bleeding will stop, as I say, once the pathological tissue has gone. I often use a 'two-sucker technique' for removing a glioblastoma—see above. But either remove it all or take only a small biopsy. To do 'a bit' is asking for a post-operative haematoma from the remaining 'purple/mauve' pathological tissue. To use a cricketing analogy, do not indulge in 'tip and run'! Do not forget hypotension especially when removing a large vascular acoustic neuroma or when facing arterial 'normal-pressure breakthrough bleeding' (NPBB). I prefer bipolar coagulation to debulk a tumour because I have damaged nerves and arteries using the ultrasonic aspirator.

Do not forget soaked cotton wool balls! I suspect the older generation of neurosurgeons never forgot cotton wool balls but these days surgeons perhaps use them less often; when left with an oozing tumour cavity, insert an unfurled cotton wool ball soaked in Ringers solution. The water adds gentle pressure while the cotton wool can be packed into the crevices. This technique is especially useful in a glioma cavity. It is also useful in meningioma surgery; having removed the bone flap over a convexity or parasagittal meningioma I often place a soaked swab or cotton wool pad over the dura and/or tumour to control the bleeding while I 'pick off' the bleeding points.

In Shakespeare's day, cobwebs were used to control bleeding (see *A Midsummer Night's Dream*). These days absorbable cellulose (Surgicel) is used and I find this very useful. I often line the tumour bed with Surgicel; it makes me feel better anyway. It is especially useful for lining a glioma cavity but be careful! All too easily one can hide bleeding points with Surgicel. I do not like to rely on Surgicel around an AVM. These fragile vessels do not respond well to Surgicel, which often disguises continued bleeding. Also Surgicel swells! Do not pack Surgicel into confined places like the pituitary fossa or spinal canal; it swells over 24 hours acting as a space-occupying lesion. Only twice have I seen an abscess form within a Surgicel-lined cavity.

There are some other tips for stopping bleeding. When removing a glioma ask the assistant to apply the diathermy to the sucker and then use the side of the end of the sucker. This is a 'poor man's laser' but it is jolly useful for performing any brain excision in a non-eloquent area. Dural bleeding is stopped well by diathermy applied to a Watson–Cheyne dissector or using bipolar coagulation. Irrigating bipolar forceps are especially useful for dissecting in an eloquent area. For bleeding bone (whether pathological or not) use wax. Get the scrub nurse to keep it warm between his or her little and ring fingers until it is needed; it is so much easier to apply warm than cold. Of course one way to stop pathological bleeding is not to produce it, especially by curbing your assistant's enthusiastic use of the sucker!

During the final stage of removing a solid haemangioblastoma, say in the brain stem, the venous return can be occluded. The tumour suddenly becomes tense, swells then ruptures. The only thing to do is to rapidly remove the tumour, which fortunately is not too difficult as this occurs only at the final stage of the dissection. However, it is a daunting experience, especially the first time it happens! The same may happen in the final stage of a hemispherectomy: this is avoided by ensuring the posterior cerebral artery is occluded before all the venous drainage is.

How do you stop bleeding from a ruptured aneurysm? Keep cool, place the sucker over the hole and by angling the sucker one can control the bleeding while you continue the dissection (one-handed) to define the main feeding artery and branches and apply a clip to the neck of the aneurysm, perhaps first applying a temporary clip to allow precise definition of the neck. Best of all is to avoid rupturing the aneurysm by careful retraction (split the Sylvian fissure rather than retract the frontal lobe), avoid two retractors, leave a layer of pia between you and the aneurysm sac, if the sac is very thin and stuck, avoid dissectors around the neck of the aneurysm (especially the part of the neck you cannot see), use temporary clips to reduce the tension in the sac if necessary (but do not over-use temporary clips as they must cause some intimal damage) and of course obtain proximal control as soon as possible as well as defining the arteries to be preserved before looking for the neck of the aneurysm.

In the section on AVMs and also on judgement, I have mentioned the problems of controlling the bleeding from AVMs. Of course the best way to avoid massive, uncontrolled bleeding from an AVM is not to operate in the first place. Yes, judgement is everything in surgery but especially with AVMs! The fine, friable vessels surrounding the nidus of an AVM can be very difficult to control. The irrigating bipolar forceps are immensely useful, I find, dealing with these vessels that all too easily stick to the forceps, tear and retract further into the brain.

Twice I have had to use a pack. The first time was operating on a vertebral haemangioma of the spine. Perhaps nowadays I would recognize it preoperatively, do a spinal angiogram, avoid surgery and give radiotherapy, as they do well with irradiation. However, the only way I could stop this bleeding was by packing and removing the pack a few days later.

For the second occasion I used the pack, see the section on pituitary tumours; the patient died from massive bleeding because of hypertension due to an unrecognized phaeochromocytoma.

Vertebral haemangiomas, to be distinguished from aneurysmal bone cysts, can be immensely vascular. Figure 38 shows such a lesion causing rapid paraplegia. Decompression of the spinal cord was necessary; the lesion's vascularity was reduced by particulate embolization, which allowed the vascular bone to be drilled carefully away. I made a point of drilling the pedicles to provide a lateral decompression before removing the lamina posteriorly. These lesions respond well to radiotherapy and if there is no cord compression it is often better to confirm the diagnosis by spinal angiography and then give radiotherapy, rather than attempting a biopsy.

Stopping arterial bleeding

Usually stopping arterial bleeding entails obliterating the artery but just occasionally it is worth trying to repair the artery. For instance I have repaired the vertebral artery on two occasions when I have damaged it between C1 and C2. Temporary clips are needed but the repair was straightforward. The same could be done for the internal carotid artery and even its large branches. If suturing is not possible then occasionally an aneurysm clip can occlude a hole in the artery.

Occasionally I have pulled a small side branch away from a larger artery. This leaves a small hole in the side of the artery, flush with the wall of the vessel. This can be quite a difficult problem, especially if the hole is on the blind side of the artery. I have found the best way to seal the hole is to use the finest bipolar forceps and apply them either side of the hole, and the coagulation is enough to seal the hole without occluding the vessel.

Otherwise, bleeding arteries have to be occluded by the usual means. Larger arteries that cannot be repaired are clipped off with aneurysm clips, while smaller vessels are coagulated. Arterial bleeding from bone (usually supplying a meningioma) is best sealed with bone wax, often applied on the back of a dissector. Sometimes arteries that cannot be occluded by a clip can be packed with Surgicel or muscle but these are methods of last resort. In general, Surgicel or muscle are not adequate for stopping arterial bleeding.

One further tip: before cutting any significant vessel (artery or vein), cut halfway across first. In this way you can check if the coagulation is sound before completing the section of a vessel. This avoids the need to chase the cut bleeding vessel ends that have retracted into the brain.

Autologous blood transfusion is useful and worth remembering. Before operating on a large and vascular aneurysmal bone cyst of the sacrum we drew off two pints of blood and then transfused the patient with his own blood at the end of the operation. This blood provides much better haemostasis.

Of course dural bleeding is often curbed by hitching the dura up to the bone with 'hitch' stitches. These are best placed through the outer layer of dura exactly at the edge of the bone. If placed away from this point

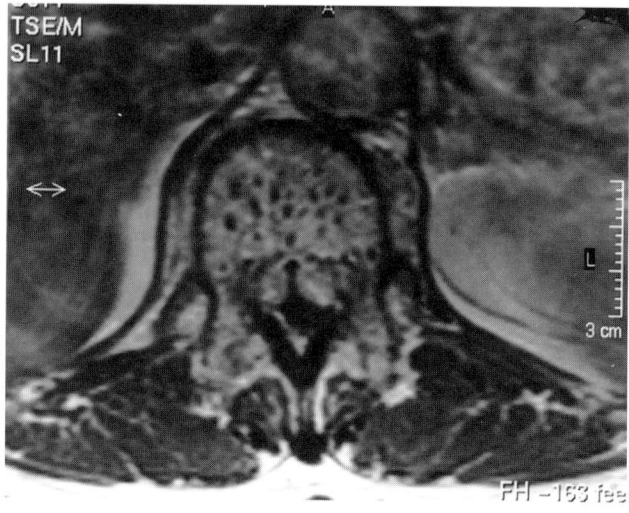

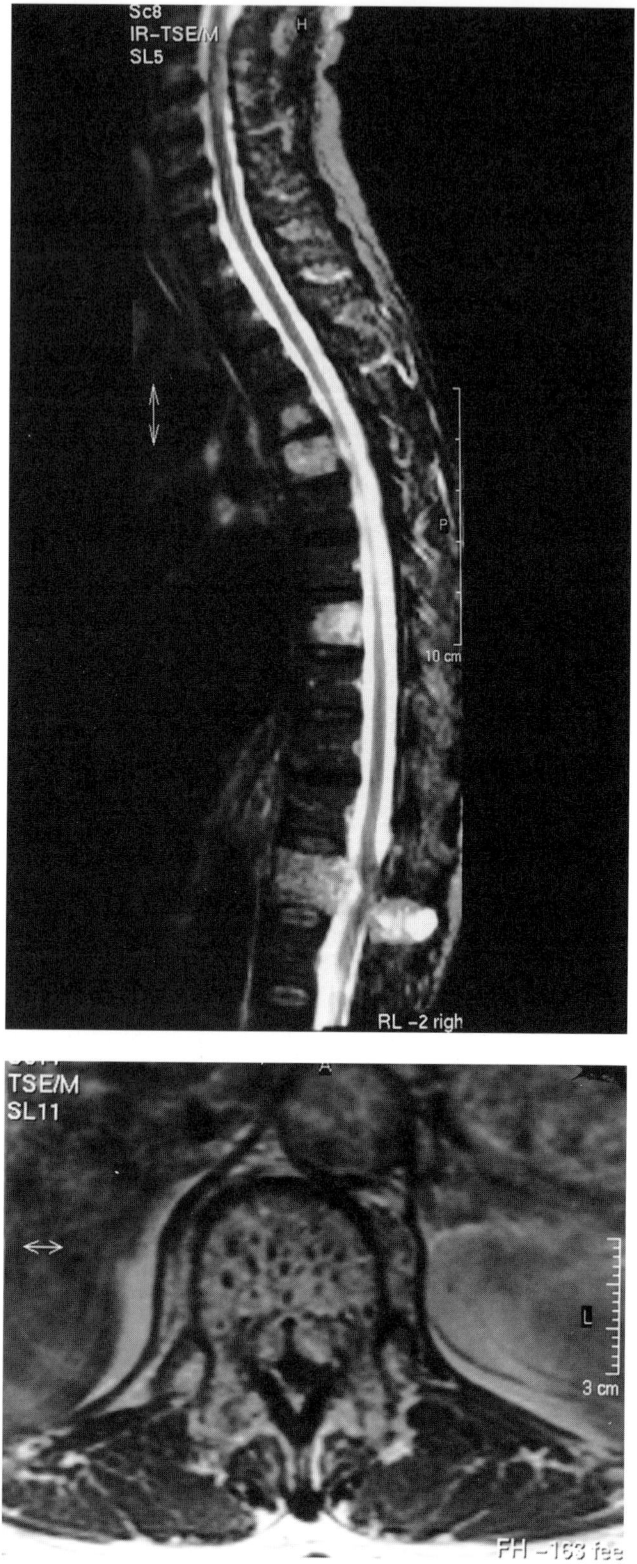

(a)

(b)

then the dura cannot be approximated closely to the bone. Often some Surgicel slipped between the bone and the dura is useful before tying the hitch stitch.

Stopping venous bleeding

Venous bleeding can always be stopped by Surgicel, pressure and patience! Best of all is to avoid it by treating epidural veins in the spinal canal with great respect or by coagulating and cutting a vein passing from the cerebellum to the transverse sinus before you avulse the vein from the side of the sinus when retracting the cerebellum! Be sure you place the Surgicel at exactly the point of bleeding; if the bleeding does not stop immediately the Surgicel is probably not correctly placed and needs repositioning. If you have avulsed a vein from a venous sinus then you will have to 'collar stud' a piece of Surgicel into the sinus with a piece inside the sinus and a component outside. To the three methods mentioned can be added another—position. In other words elevate the head to reduce the venous pressure. Even better is to position the patient to avoid a high venous pressure, hence my liking for the sitting or reclining position when appropriate. One tip: after spinal surgery a suction drain may fill rather alarmingly with (venous) blood. If this happens it usually means the suction drain is adjacent to a vein. Switch the drain off and turn the patient onto his or her side to reduce the abdominal compression and hence the high epidural venous pressure. I have never seen a significant haematoma develop switching the suction drain off. By the way, never leave a suction drain in the spine when the dura has been opened. I have seen CSF rapidly sucked into the drain producing intracerebral haemorrhage and death.

Of course other standard methods will stop venous bleeding: using the

Fig. 38 (a,b) MRI scans to show multiple vertebral haemangiomas, one of which was causing spinal cord compression. The axial scan shows encroachment of the spinal canal. The sagittal scan shows the multiple lesions and the post-operative decompression. The patient's paraplegia recovered but she became constipated and nauseated in the post-operative period. We found an elevated serum calcium. An (unrelated) parathyroid tumour was found and removed. Do routine calcium levels in women over 40 years of age! The patient later received low-dose radiotherapy to the vertebral haemangioma; these curious tumours are very radiosensitive.

diathermy on a sucker or Watson–Cheyne dissector is useful. I do not know why there is a high venous pressure in the diploic veins with raised intracranial pressure (RICP) but once the pressure is reduced this venous bleeding will be reduced.

Sometimes it will be necessary to suture a venous sinus. It is useful to first apply a mosquito forceps, which will crimp the edges; these will stay approximated when the forceps is removed and allow the suture to be inserted without undue bleeding.

One last tip: veins when coagulated shorten. Therefore when you coagulate a vein, release your retraction slightly otherwise the vein may pull out of the sinus it is entering. This may occur, for instance, coagulating the petrosal vein entering the sigmoid sinus. Much better to avoid that!

Just occasionally it can be difficult to decide if one has found a chronic subdural haematoma or venous blood. I saw one young neurosurgeon nearly exsanguinate a patient with a chronic subdural haematoma. He had entered a vein and not the subdural space. The way to avoid this is to carefully open the dura and identify the subdural membrane before formally opening it.

How to preserve cranial nerves

The only way to preserve the function of a cranial nerve is not to touch it! Thus, when removing an acoustic neuroma, avoid touching the seventh nerve or the cochlear nerve. When removing a suprasellar meningioma debulk the tumour at a distance from the optic nerve before 'rolling' the immediately adjacent tumour away from the nerve. When drilling bone away drill to the cortex then gently 'crack' the remaining bone away with a dissector. Avoid blind dissection with dissectors along the optic foramen or internal auditory meatus; in other words obtain the best possible exposure before dissecting tumour away from the nerve. Use the least retraction needed. Avoid bipolar coagulation near the nerve or if necessary to coagulate, use irrigating bipolar forceps. Use frequent irrigation to cool the tissues down. Use sharp dissection rather than blunt dissection.

There is one cranial nerve that seems to stop working for a while whenever it meets fresh air; that is the third nerve. One only has to look at it for it to stop working for about 3 months but fortunately it usually recovers.

Do not rely on preserving an optic nerve which is severely compressed as it passes through an optic foramen. However gentle and patient I am removing the surrounding bone of the optic foramen I have often failed to preserve the remaining vision in that eye and one must warn the patient of this difficulty pre-operatively.

Equally I would personally be loath to advise an operation to preserve hearing in patients with bilateral acoustic neuromas. Some experts may claim to be able to do this with sufficient certainty so they could advise such a patient, deaf in one ear to undergo removal of an acoustic neuroma in the remaining, hearing, ear. I cannot and would not advise it. I would recommend waiting. If the hearing was deteriorating rapidly I would seriously consider stereotactic irradiation. I have tried intracapsular removal of the tumour in these circumstances but have still damaged the hearing. The problem is we need 'on-line' monitoring of hearing, which as yet we do not have. Fortunately brain-stem 'cochlear'-type implants may in the future allow hearing even after the cochlear nerve has been sacrificed. Neurofibromatosis Type II is a devastatingly awful disease (if only because other members of the family have witnessed its awfulness before it affects them) and I have learned to avoid surgery in these afflicted patients if at all possible and only advise an operation when the symptoms demand it.

Tips on operating within the ventricles

I have two personal rules. The first is to place a pattie in the ventricle as soon as the ventricle is entered to prevent blood seeping in and filling the whole ventricular system. Secondly, if in doubt, leave a ventricular catheter in the ventricle before coming out. Leave it (switched off) for 48 hours just to make sure one can immediately treat any acute hydrocephalus that may develop post-operatively. I am very fond of the trans-callosal approach to the lateral and third ventricles. Place your 'parasagittal' incision at least 1 cm over the midline to the opposite side so you will always have the dural opening as near the sagittal sinus as possible (see Figure 12(b)). Failure to do this will make the operation difficult! Place the posterior extent of the bone flap at, and no further back than, the coronal suture. Aim in line with the external auditory meatus and you will find the foramen of Munro! Always fenestrate the septum pellicidum so that if a shunt is needed only a unilateral shunt will be required. Bilateral shunts cause trouble! The choroid plexus will tell you that you are in the ventricle and if you follow that, you will find the foramen of Munro and will also be able to tell which ventricle you are in, the left or the right!

Of course, absolute haemostasis is essential: do not leave bits of Surgicel floating around, although I often use Surgicel when required; do not, of course, use hydrogen peroxide anywhere near the ventricles (I only use hydrogen peroxide after I have closed the dura and then only when I have done a hemispherectomy creating an extradural space); finally, refill the ventricles with warm Ringers solution before closing the dura. If the patient does not wake up rapidly following the cessation of the anaesthetic do a CT scan to make sure there is no intraventricular clot. Do not wait for overt clinical deterioration. This is a good general rule after any neurosurgical intracranial procedure.

I leave you with three other tips. First, do not leave an external drain in the ventricle longer than 5 days. The infection rate increases markedly after 5 days. Secondly, when removing a colloid cyst in the third ventricle do not worry about leaving some of the cyst wall over the origin of the internal cerebral veins. I always do this to make sure I do not damage these vital veins and have never had a recurrence. Curiously, textbooks do not mention this, nor do they stress that you may have to look for the colloid cyst from both right and left sides (via the fenestrated septum pellucidum) to find it. It can be quite difficult to find sometimes. Finally, to gain access to a large third ventricle lesion you need to coagulate the choroid plexus to gently gain access to the third ventricle. This entails coagulating and cutting the thalamo-striate vein. It is my experience that it is safe to do this but I ensure cutting this well away from its junction with the internal cerebral vein.

Should you do a post-operative computed tomography scan?

I refer to the CT scan rather than to the MRI scan because CT scans show blood, and anyway patients have too much metal applied to them in the post-operative phase to allow an MRI scan.

The answer varies. Yes, of course, do a CT scan if the patient wakes up and then deteriorates. If the patient deteriorates quickly it may be better to take them back to theatre without a CT scan. Sometimes I do an immediate post-operative CT scan with the patient still anaesthetized, if I am worried about a haematoma after perhaps removing a large, difficult AVM. More difficult is when the patient is slow to wake up from the anaesthetic. I have no doubt that in these circumstances it is better to do a CT scan sooner rather than later. I have had four patients who have developed contralateral cerebellar haemorrhagic infarcts after a pterional craniotomy; the patient who made a good recovery was the one reoperated on quickly with removal of the infarct. Why does it happen? I believe the rapid evacuation of CSF allows the most dependent (opposite) cerebellar lobe to 'fall' on its own venous drainage, perhaps kinking the draining vein or veins. So look carefully at the posterior fossa after a pterional craniotomy! One other tip: after a temporal lobe operation ask the radiologist to angle the scan gantry in the line of the temporal lobe. Routine scans cut across the temporal lobe but it will be much easier to see a post-operative haematoma if the scan is performed in the line of the temporal lobe.

Repair of cerebrospinal fluid leaks

CSF is remarkable stuff. It is also remarkably difficult to confine to the central nervous system, which is a very good reason for never operating on Tarlov cysts of the lumbo-sacral sac. Another reason for not operating on Tarlov cysts is that it does not stop the patient's pain, in my experience.

CSF leaks are seen after trans-sphenoidal surgery, skull base surgery, acoustic neuroma and other cerebello-pontine angle operations as well as spinal operations. I have a few observations. The first is that small holes in the arachnoid cause many more problems than large holes because they act as a one-way valve. CSF escapes during a transient rise of pressure and thus a collection of CSF may develop under very high pressure and even rupture the overlying skin.

It follows that to repair a CSF leak the surgeon has to find the exact point of leakage through the arachnoid. It is far more effective to place a fascial graft on the pia side of the arachnoid so that the pressure of the brain and CSF closes the hole even more securely with elevation of the intracranial pressure. Indeed, a well repaired hole will withstand a valsalva manoeuvre without the dural graft being sutured. When repairing a CSF leak through the diaphragma sella of a pituitary fossa it pays to 'collar stud' the hole by passing a piece of fascia lata through the hole so that it sits on top of the diaphragma. The second principle I find useful is to obliterate the adjacent dead space. I find a pedicle muscle graft particularly effective after spinal or skull base surgery but clearly this is not feasible after trans-sphenoidal pituitary surgery or acoustic neuroma surgery. Figure 39 illustrates the principles I use for repairing spinal leaks. In this situation I insert the graft between the arachnoid and the dura, so that the dural sutures do not penetrate the arachnoid and once again the elevated CSF pressure will seal the hole even more securely.

When stopping intracranial leaks, 5 days or so of spinal drainage does often seem helpful by reducing the intracranial pressure, thus stemming the flow through the 'fistula' but if there is a distal obstruction in the form of a

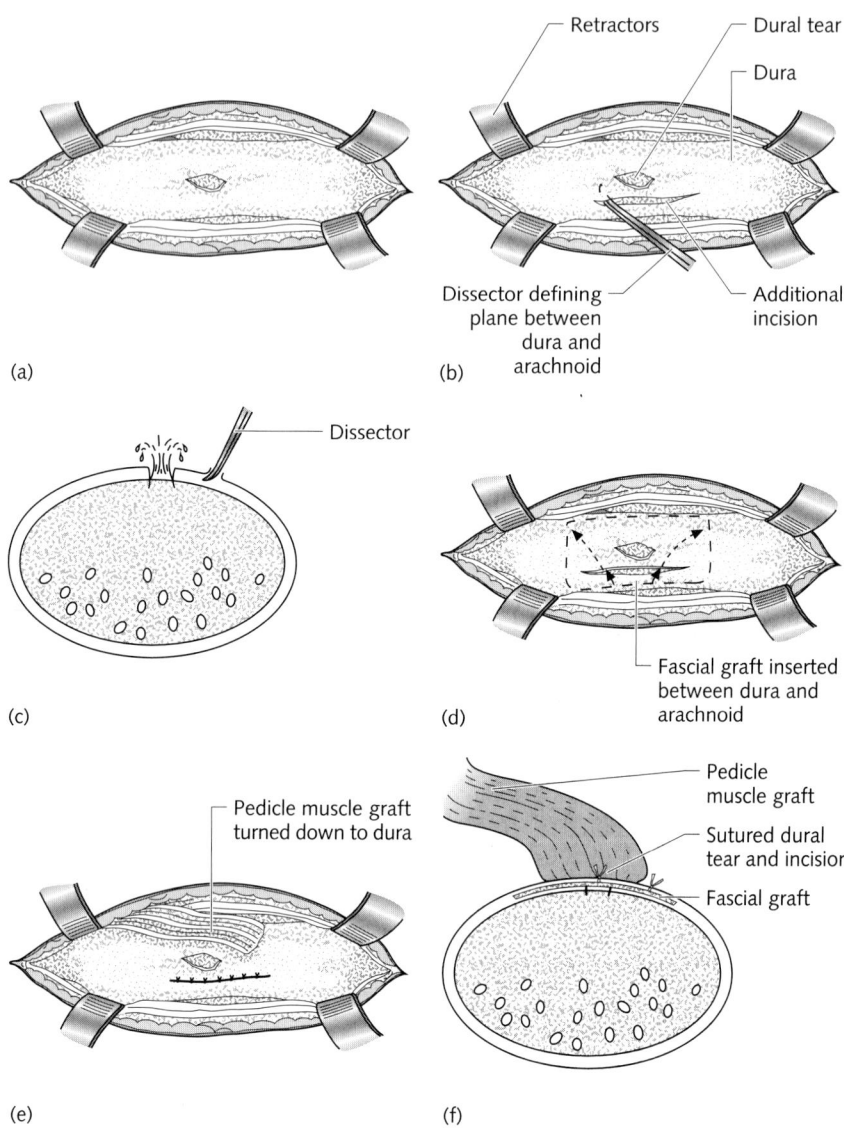

(a)

(b)

Retractors

Dural tear

Dura

Dissector defining plane between dura and arachnoid

Additional incision

Dissector

(c)

(d)

Fascial graft inserted between dura and arachnoid

(e)

Pedicle muscle graft turned down to dura

(f)

Pedicle muscle graft

Sutured dural tear and incision

Fascial graft

Fig. 39 (a–f) Diagrams to show a method of repairing spinal CSF leaks. The principles are first, to place the fascia on the subdural side of the dura so the intracranial and intraspinal CSF pressure presses the graft against the dura; and secondly, it is important to eliminate the extradural dead space.

communicating hydrocephalus, then insertion of a shunt may well be necessary before the CSF leak can be stopped (see Table 6, p. 58).

Pterional craniotomy

This is a frequently performed craniotomy for lesions of the anterior cranial fossa, sella and suprasellar region as well as the middle and indeed posterior cranial fossae. It is the usual 'aneurysm flap'. It is desirable to avoid damage to the facial nerve branch supplying the frontalis muscle and although there are various solutions to this, I feel comfortable with the one I have developed (Figure 40). Splitting the Sylvian fissure is an important part of the operation and I will describe a few tips I have learned over the years.

The pterional approach is simply a method to get to the floor of the anterior cranial fossa as signified by the frontozygomatic suture. The scalp flap is placed behind the hairline of sufficient length to hinge down to this suture just behind the eyebrow. To preserve the facial nerves I avoid cutting the pericranium and temporalis muscle too low down but incise these structures a centimetre or so above the frontozygomatic suture and then undermine and elevate these tissues off the bone. This allows the desired exposure of the frontozygomatic suture with preservation of the branches of the facial nerve. I still prefer the Gigli saw because it is safer, particularly when the dura is densely adherent to the bone as in the elderly, and also because the bone cut is thinner, which allows the bone flap to be replaced more accurately without the need for wiring. I use the retained pericranium to suture the bone flap into place and fill the burr holes with the retained bone dust. I am amazed that devascularized, free bone flaps do not often become infected; it is extremely rare for them to need removal despite my initial fears. After the flap has been removed I nibble the sphenoid wing away to expose the floor of the anterior cranial fossa. When operating for an anterior communicating artery aneurysm it is helpful to remove the bevel at the inner table of the skull along the eyebrow to increase the exposure by a few millimetres. It is unusual to enter the frontal sinus but if so then I use a temporalis fascial graft to suture over the exposed frontal sinus, the graft being placed between the pericranium above and the dura below. It is important to stop any extradural ooze at this stage; once the dura is opened and CSF aspirated, the dura will tend to fall away from the bone and further bleeding will inevitably occur which can be an irritating distraction once the operating microscope has been introduced.

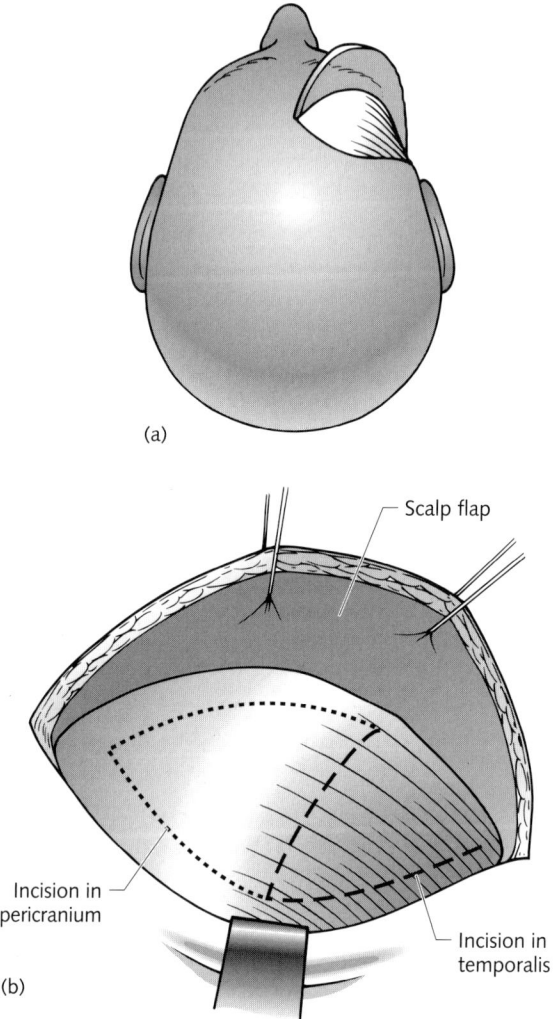

(a)

Scalp flap

Incision in
pericranium

Incision in
temporalis

(b)

Fig. 40 (a–d) Diagrams to show the author's method of pterional craniotomy to preserve
the facial nerve branches to the eyebrow and forehead. At the end of the procedure the
bone flap (with attached pericranium) is resutured into position and the triangular muscle
flap resutured to the remaining temporalis muscle and to the cuff of temporalis muscle left
on the temporal crest of the bone flap. (*Continued*)

Splitting the Sylvian fissure

Splitting the Sylvian fissure atraumatically can be one of the most difficult
technical exercises in neurosurgery. Sometimes it is delightfully easy but at
other times, especially when carrying out early aneurysm surgery, it can be

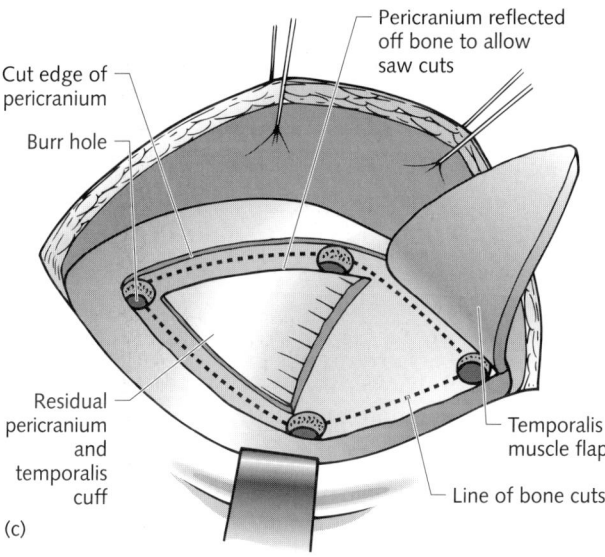

Pericranium reflected off bone to allow saw cuts

Cut edge of pericranium

Burr hole

Residual pericranium and temporalis cuff

Temporalis muscle flap

Line of bone cuts

(c)

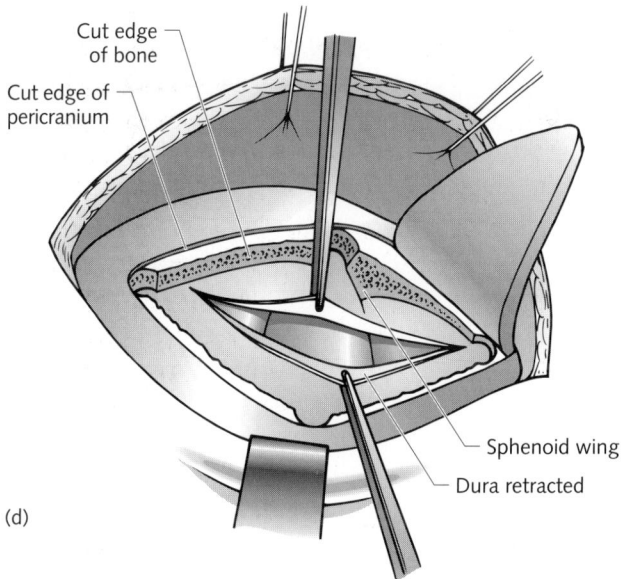

Cut edge of bone

Cut edge of pericranium

Sphenoid wing

Dura retracted

(d)

Fig. 40 (*Continued*)

extremely difficult. I have two tips. The temporal lobe overhangs the Sylvian fissure so having cut the arachnoid on the frontal lobe side of the Sylvian vein I recommend swinging the microscope so that it is directed laterally, looking, in effect, under the opercula of the temporal lobe. These opercula can be held upwards by using the sucker held in the left hand. The best way I find to obtain the correct plane between the two lobes is to find a cortical artery on the frontal lobe side and trace it into the depths of the Sylvian fissure (Figure 41). It is often surprisingly easy to do this. Once one has created a tunnel then one can gently extend the tunnel by parting the fissure with the bipolar forceps from the depths, superficially. Obviously if one is operating on a middle cerebral aneurysm one avoids dissecting the fissure deeply. In these circumstances I cut the arachnoid and gently and cautiously work my way down to the internal carotid artery in order to get proximal control. When splitting the fissure one constantly has to debate which vessel belongs to which lobe. The anterior temporal branch of the middle cerebral artery is a constant landmark in the proximal Sylvian fissure. At this point the overlying arachnoid becomes tough and there is often a Sylvian vein traversing the fissure, which needs coagulating and cutting. Fortunately, it is extremely rare to get haemorrhagic infarction following sacrifice of the Sylvian veins (unlike the vein of Labbé) but obviously one does not want to sacrifice any vein or artery unnecessarily, however small. The advantage of splitting the Sylvian fissure is that this parts the frontal from the temporal lobe obviating the need to retract the frontal lobe. This also allows early identification of the internal carotid artery when for instance, operating on suprasellar tumours such as meningiomas. If the frontal lobe is retracted upwards away from the anterior cranial fossa there is more chance of rupturing an aneurysm sac, particularly if it is an internal carotid aneurysm or an anterior communicating artery aneurysm directed anteriorly and adherent to the optic chiasm.

Meningiomas

The traditional principles for treating a meningioma are to remove the centre of the tumour and then to gently tease the capsule away from the surrounding brain. With the advent of the operating microscope and the ability to operate through a narrow exposure, I would stress the advantage of early obliteration of the tumour blood supply. If for instance, the tumour can be detached from its origin from the anterior cranial fossa at an early stage of the operation, the subsequent dissection from the surrounding structures will be much facilitated. Of course, finding and maintaining the correct plane between tumour and brain is crucial, as with all surgery, but especially for

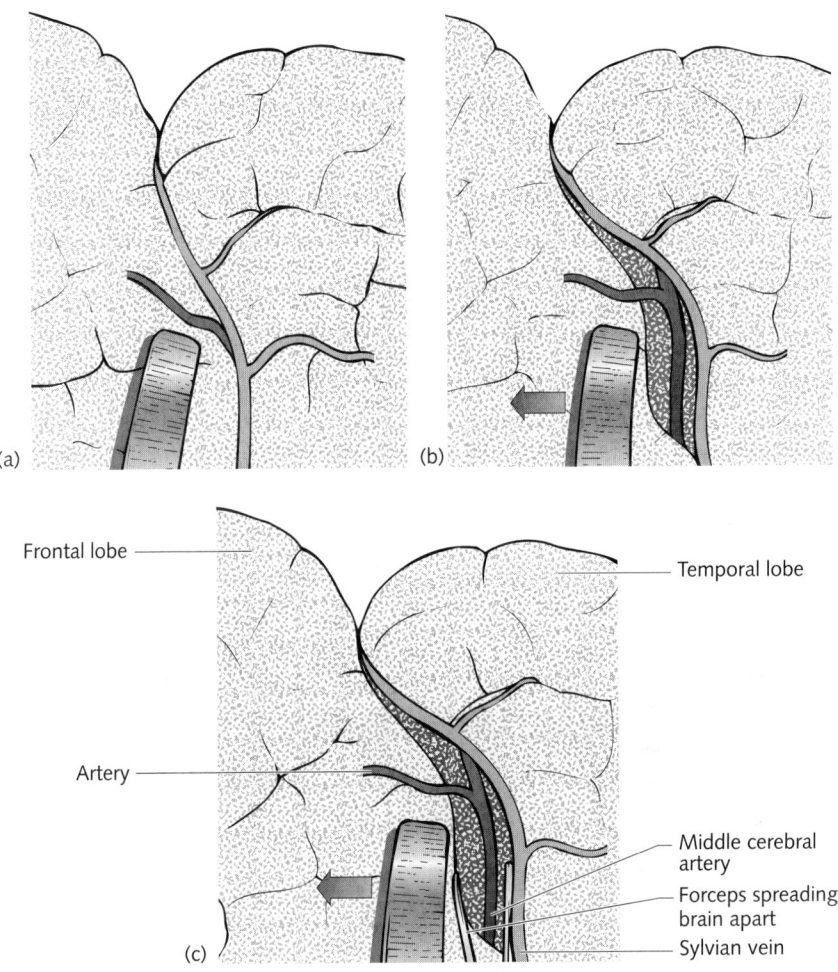

(a)

(b)

Frontal lobe —

— Temporal lobe

Artery —

— Middle cerebral artery

— Forceps spreading brain apart

(c)

— Sylvian vein

Fig. 41 (a–c) Diagrams to show splitting of the Sylvian fissure: this can be remarkably difficult or remarkably easy. I have found the best method is to find a cortical artery and trace this into the Sylvian fissure, 'tunnelling' along the artery until one finds the major middle cerebral artery or its branches. Then one opens the fissure from this tunnel proceeding from the depth to superficially and proximally. Obviously if there is a middle cerebral artery aneurysm then one avoids dissecting deeply into the fissure until one gets proximal control of the main middle cerebral artery.

operations for meningiomas and acoustic neuromas. The scan in Figure 42 demonstrates a left parasagittal meningioma causing focal motor and sensory epilepsy of the foot. The scan shows a thin rim of low density on the T2 image. At operation the tumour was soft and could be gently dissected away leaving intact cortex lining the tumour bed. Post-operatively (Figure 43) there was no neurological deficit. I am certain if this tumour had a harder

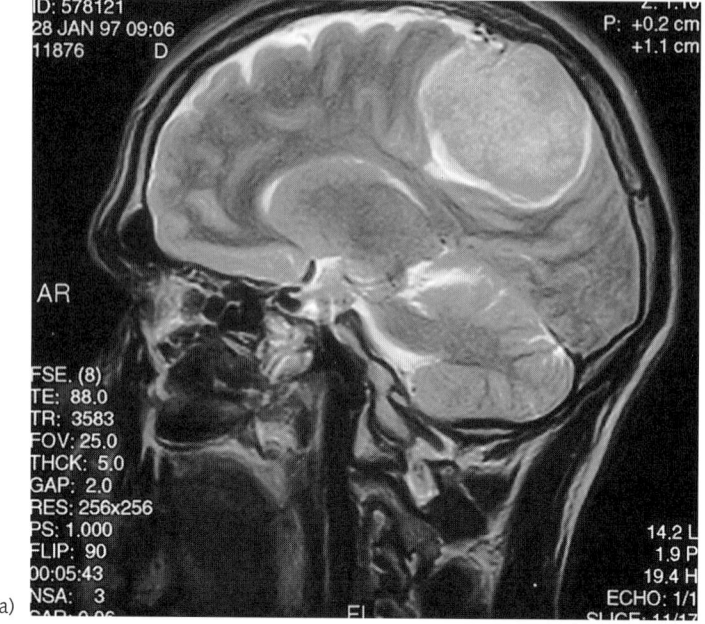

(a)

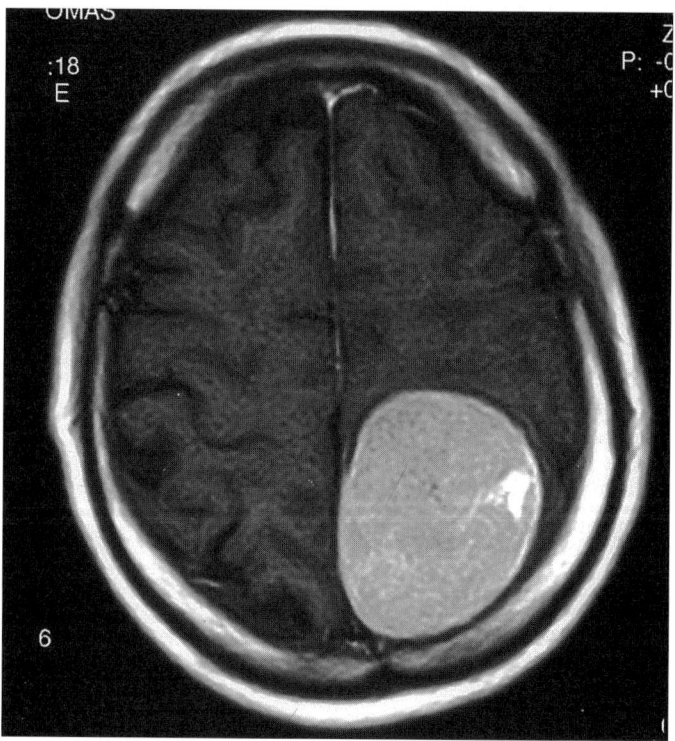

(b)

Fig. 42 Parasagittal meningioma. The patient presented with focal motor epilepsy of the right leg. The MRI scan shows a clear margin between tumour and brain. The cortex was in fact intact and not ulcerated by the tumour. Dissecting in the correct (subdural) plane allowed the tumour to be completely removed without neurological deficit. See Figure 43.

consistency it would have ulcerated through the cortex causing a greater neurological deficit pre- and post-operatively. Although soft tumours, of similar consistency to brain, are more difficult to dissect from the brain, they do tend to be associated with less damage to the surrounding brain. I believe this is true for acoustic neuromas as well. When operating on a parasagittal meningioma one is operating on the draining veins as much as anything and the preservation of these determine the quality of the result. If it is necessary

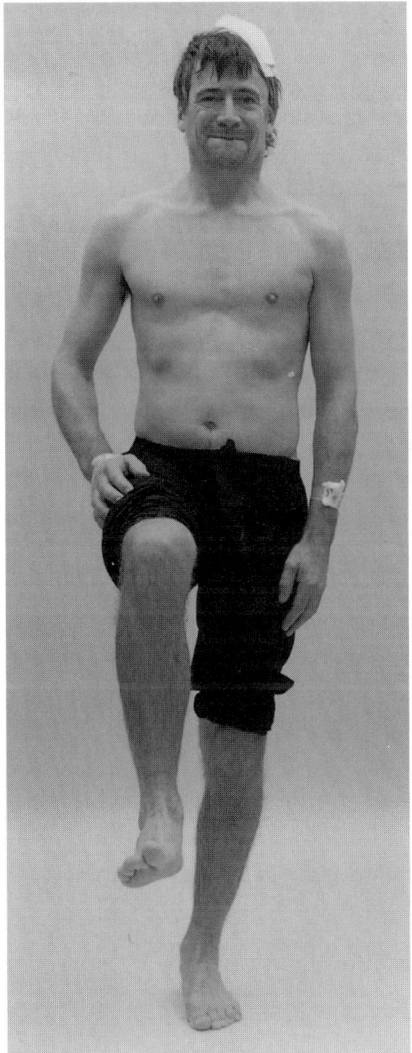
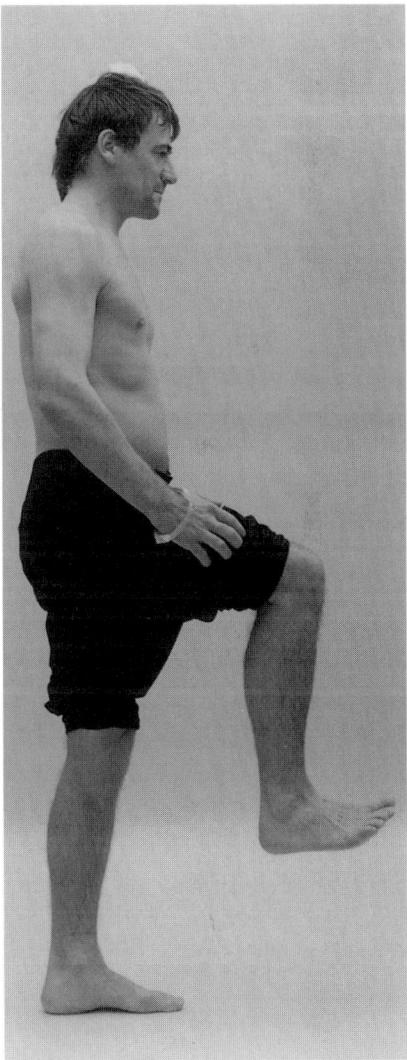

Fig. 43 The patient in Figure 42 showing power of dorsiflexion of the right foot, 2 days post-operatively.

to open the lateral edge of the sagittal sinus to remove tumour, I find it useful to use a series of mosquito forceps. These 'crimp' the edge of the sinus and allow the surgeon to run a continuous suture along the sinus after removing the forceps one by one.

Petroclinoid meningiomas are difficult but having tried various approaches I prefer the 'Malis' approach. Malis describes a combined middle and posterior fossa approach, removing as much of the mastoid process to expose the superior petrosal sinus, the transverse sinus and the vein of Labbé. The transverse sinus is tied off between the superior petrosal sinus and the vein of Labbé. This section through the transverse sinus is continued forward and medially parallel to the superior petrosal sinus to the tentorial notch. This allows the temporal lobe, the tentorium and the transverse sinus together with the vein of Labbé to be elevated. I have learned to treat the vein of Labbé with the greatest respect and this approach respects the integrity of the vein better than any other approach. Of course angiography (with ipsilateral jugular compression) is necessary pre-operatively to determine venous outflow and the safety of tying off the transverse sinus. If this is not possible then the surgeon has a choice of working either side of the sinus and cutting the tentorium or tying off the superior petrosal sinus to allow posterior retraction against the sigmoid and transverse sinuses. I prefer the latter because it still gets you where you want to be although with less exposure and more danger to the vein of Labbé. One piece of advice: if you know you cannot take the lateral (or sigmoid) sinus my advice is leave the bone over the sinus intact so as not to run the risk of damaging it. I did damage the sinus once in these circumstances and was forced to tie off the sinus. I abandoned the operation and to my relief the patient was completely unaffected. Six months later I removed her large petroclinoid meningioma without complications.

I have a few suggestions when carrying out this procedure. First, I 'flap' the pericranium and muscles over the middle and posterior fossae so that when coming out I can get a good watertight closure. Secondly, before committing oneself to any particular place to section the transverse sinus, open the temporal dura and carefully trace the draining veins into the transverse sinus. These can be very variable and sometimes one cannot safely tie the transverse sinus between the superior petrosal sinus and vein(s) of Labbé. Once I had to cut the superior petrosal sinus and tie off the sigmoid sinus instead of the transverse sinus. I find it easier to cut the tentorium looking at it from above than below: it is easier to cut parallel to the petrous bone (and avoid the otherwise troublesome superior petrosal sinus) and to avoid the fourth nerve. Although Malis prefers the sitting position, I much prefer the patient lying on the back, with the head turned to the opposite direction and tilted about 20° to bring the sloping tentorium to a more horizontal position. I always prepare a thigh, for invariably I need a fascial graft to close the dura and fat to fill the dead space left by the removal of the mastoid process. I agree with Malis that it is an immensely useful flap for lesions in front of the brain stem or straddling the middle and posterior fossa. Once the tent is cut one comes down on the fifth nerve exposing this structure better than any other approach.

I have been through an aggressive phase removing skull base cavernous sinus meningiomas but I have been impressed by the morbidity of such surgery, which combined with the rather frequent inability to achieve a complete tumour removal inclines me usually to advise removal of the easily and safely removable component of the tumour and rely on stereotactic radiosurgery to suppress further growth of the remainder. One has to accept that however aggressive and determined one is, some skull base meningiomas are impossible to remove totally.

Finally, remember the last thing attached to a meningioma is always a blood vessel! However tempting it may be to pull out the last remaining lump of tumour, don't!

Foramen magnum meningiomas: postero-lateral inferior approach

Anterior or lateral foramen magnum meningiomas do require a postero-lateral approach (George & Lot, 1995, see Further reading). I find it best to make a midline incision, which then turns along the superior nuchal line and if necessary down the mastoid process along the posterior border of the sternomastoid muscle. 'If necessary' means if the vertebral artery is surrounded by tumour and needs mobilization along the C1 transverse process and posterior arch. In my experience this is unusual. It is useful to expose the occipital condyle (this is obvious once the joint capsule has been entered) and then drill off the postero-medial part of the condyle up to the hypoglossal canal and the adjacent skull base to the groove of the sigmoid sinus. The extra exposure is useful for the 'inferior' approach to the tumour.

This is one aspect of these tumours that has not been emphasized in any publication that I have read and I believe deserves to be. Much emphasis is placed on the far lateral approach with the inference that one has to approach laterally. Actually I think one needs to approach these tumours posteriorly, laterally and inferiorly. If one studies Figure 44 one can see that these meningiomas grow up pushing into the cerebellum and brain stem. As mentioned earlier, one wants to remove the tumour in the opposite direction to which it grows to allow its delivery in the most atraumatic fashion. I therefore strongly recommend the sitting position. Do not over-flex the head otherwise the already stretched brain stem will be further bow strung over the tumour. By removing the postero-medial superior part of the occipital condyle one can obtain a more inferior approach. The other important point is the angle made by the clivus is about 45° (parallel to the straight sinus) so that if the head and body is flexed and rotated forward by 45° the clivus is conveniently horizontal. This allows the surgeon to detach the tumour from the clivus with minimal retraction, so devascularizing the tumour early. This produces an avascular tumour, very considerably aiding gentle dissection of the tumour from the surrounding nerves, especial-

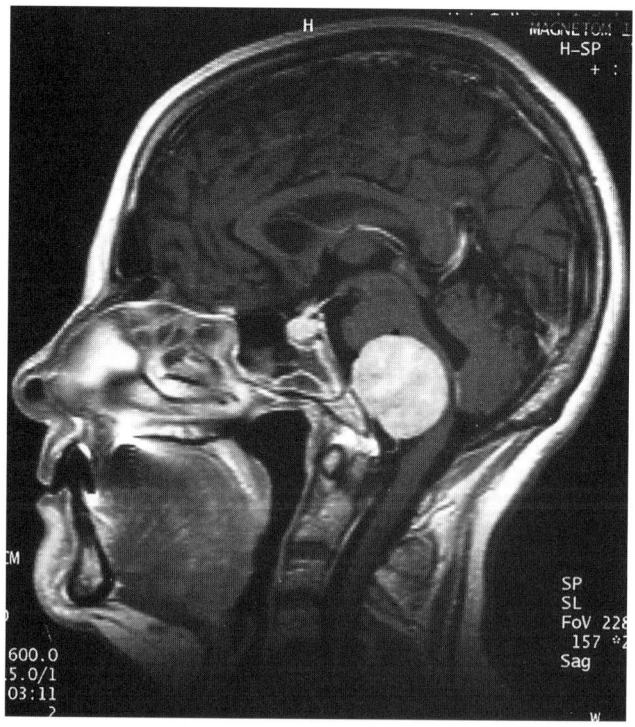

(a)

Fig. 44 (a–c) Pre-operative MRI and CT scans of a 60-year-old woman with a 7-year history of dysphagia and more recently truncal ataxia and choking. The scans show the tumour arising from the anterior and right side of the foramen magnum. A postero-lateral inferior approach was carried out and the tumour was easily and atraumatically removed. (*Continued*)

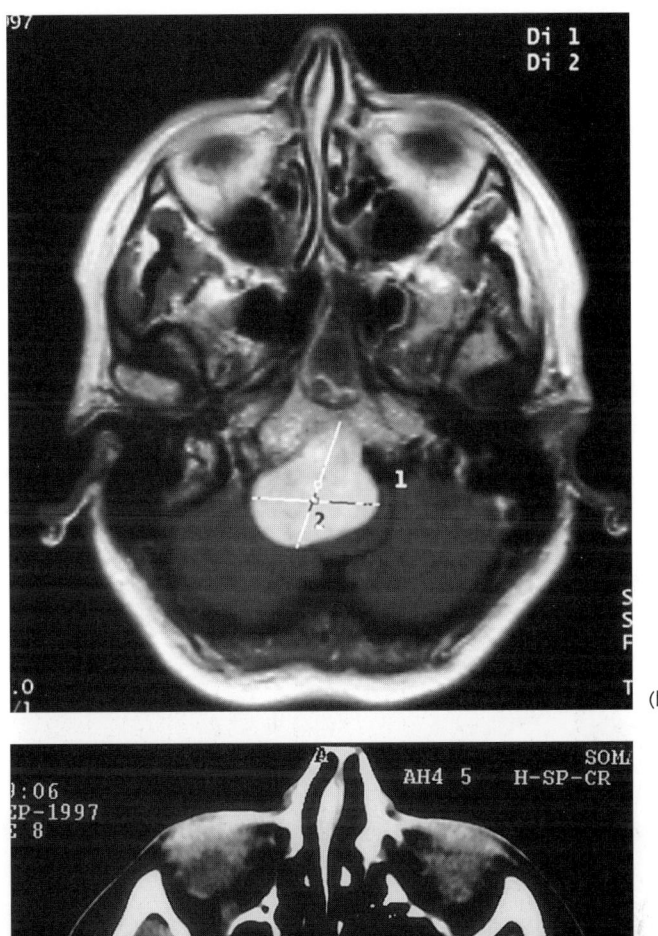

(b)

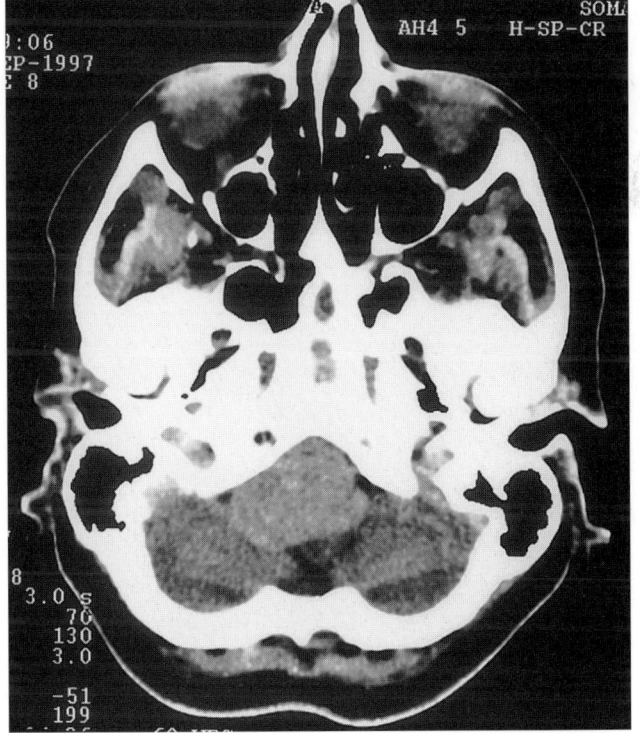

(c)

Fig. 44 (*Continued*)

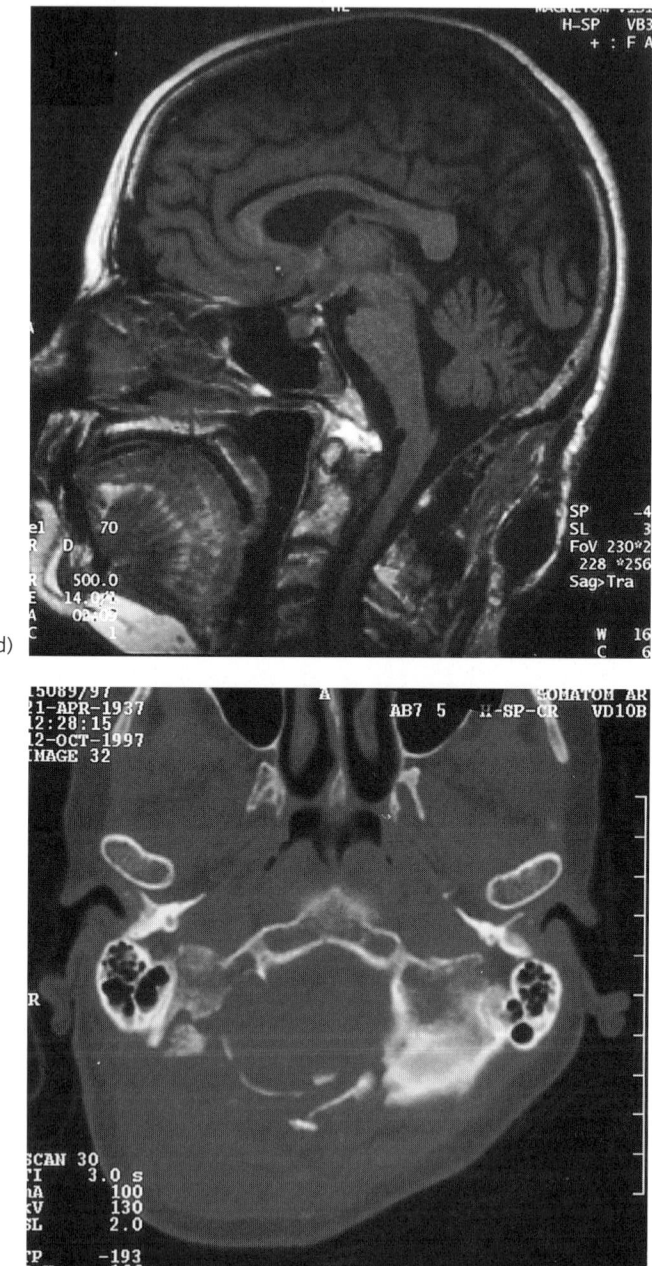

(d)

(e)

Fig. 44 (*Continued*) (d,e) The post-operative MRI and CT scans showing the extent of bone removal. The CT scan shows the jugular process of the occipital bone has been partially removed (and the posterior part of the occipital condyle). The fragments of bone seen on the CT scan were replaced at the end of the operation to reconstitute the occipital bone.

ly the vagal group. With the patient in the sitting position, gravity aids the delivery of the tumour from the brain stem and surrounding cranial nerves and arteries. I thoroughly recommend this inferior emphasis. In other words, concentrate on getting underneath the tumour rather than just lateral to it. Do try it. See Figure 44.

I (and a patient) have had one traumatic experience with these tumours; the patient had severe dysphagia and a large, exactly midline anterior foramen magnum meningioma, which was calcified. I took this out from a right postero-lateral approach. It was so hard I could only use a scalpel blade. I removed this tumour completely but post-operatively she was paralysed from the neck down but with intact sensation. Fortunately she made a complete recovery, but only after 6 months. I presume the manipulations bruised the pyramidal tracts (I was sure I had not damaged the anterior spinal arteries). If faced with that situation again I would stage the procedure, removing the right half only from the right side and the left half at a later stage using a left postero-lateral inferior approach.

Spinal meningiomas

An anteriorly placed spinal meningioma represents the exception to the rule concerned with detaching the tumour from its blood supply. The spinal cord may be tightly stretched over such a tumour and the slightest manipulation of the stretched cord may cause cord damage. This statement arises from a bitter experience. I removed an anteriorly placed meningioma at C2. I approached this laterally and removed the meningioma without directly touching the cord. I was devastated when the patient woke up quadriplegic and I can only surmise that the manipulations necessary to detach the tumour from its dural blood supply caused this damage. Fortunately the patient made a good recovery over a 6-month period. After that experience I have always debulked the tumour before detaching the tumour from its dural origin once the stretched cord has been decompressed.

Temporal lobe surgery

Of all the intracranial procedures, I think operations on the temporal lobe are the least well performed. The reason for this is insufficient appreciation of the anatomy medial to the temporal lobe. Figure 45 illustrates the structures seen and I would particularly emphasize the three vessels—the posterior cerebral artery, the anterior choroidal artery and the basal vein of

Rosenthal (and the optic tract)—all lying medial to the temporal lobe against the mid-brain, covered by a layer of arachnoid. When carrying out temporal lobe operations by any route this layer of arachnoid and the choroid plexus must be kept intact. The arachnoid can only be cut lateral to the free edge of the tentorium. Furthermore there is an important sulcus between the hippocampus and the parahippocampal gyrus. This is called the hippocampal sulcus and receives branches of the anterior choroidal and posterior cerebral arteries supplying the hippocampus and amygdala, the latter being quite a vascular structure. When removing the hippocampus it is necessary to coagulate and cut these branches running into the hippocampal sulcus taking care not to 'button hole' the anterior choroidal artery. Only when this sulcus has been coagulated and cut can the surgeon remove the hippocampus and amygdala from the all-important layer of arachnoid covering the mid-brain and the three vessels mentioned above.

There are two approaches to the temporal lobe. The classical Falconer temporal lobectomy, removing the amygdala and hippocampus with the temporal lobe and secondly the Yasargil amygdalohippocampectomy through the Sylvian fissure. The lobectomy is performed when widespread

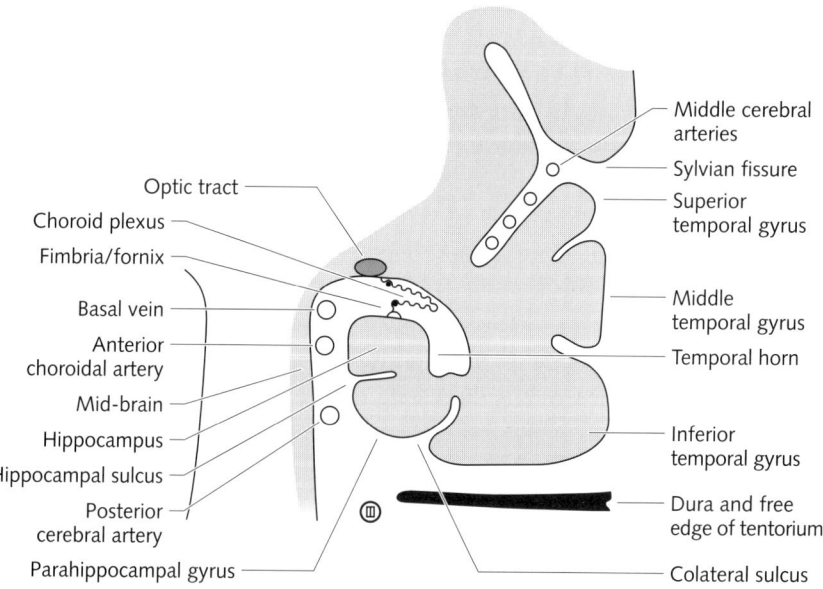

Fig. 45 The anatomy of the medial temporal lobe to emphasize the three vessels against the mid-brain and the importance of not cutting the arachnoid except lateral to the free edge of the tentorium.

pathology exists in the temporal lobe while the advantage of the Yasargil approach is the preservation of the visual fields. This operation is only appropriate for more localized pathology affecting the anterior and medial parts of the temporal lobe (see Further reading).

Classical temporal lobectomy

As there are rather few clear descriptions of the operative technique in standard texts, I will expand on the technique I use. Usually a 6-cm excision is carried out. Six centimetres represents a compromise. More than 6 cm usually produces a hemianopia whereas 6 cm or less produces an inevitable quadrantinopia, although 10% of patients may develop a hemianopia. I prefer a question-mark incision starting in front of the tragus at the zygomatic arch curling back over the pinna before passing forwards. It is important not to make the flap too long and narrow, otherwise the vascularity of the distal part of the flap will be endangered. A circumferential fascial incision allows the temporalis muscle and bone flap to be retracted well away from the temporal pole region allowing a good exposure of this otherwise rather difficult to expose area. After the dura is opened the 6-cm point is measured from the tip of the temporal pole using a brain needle (Figure 46). Two particular landmarks are used when carrying out the lobectomy. First the temporal horn of the ventricle and secondly the free edge of the tentorium leading into the wing of the sphenoid. The temporal horn is found by making an incision at the 6-cm mark (or less if the vein of Labbé is sited there) through the middle temporal gyrus. The horn is found at 4-cm depth and is confirmed by noting the presence of choroid plexus. This incision is deepened further at right angles to the cortex to find the edge of the tentorium by dissecting through the inferior aspect of the temporal lobe. The surgeon then moves to the Sylvian fissure coagulating and cutting the pia-arachnoid along the line of the fissure eventually finding the sphenoid wing (Figure 46). The Sylvian veins at this point are, if possible, preserved and the incision prolonged to meet the anterior insertion of the free edge of the tentorium. I find it useful to gently elevate the temporal lobe at this point to identify the whole extent of the edge of the tentorium in order to coagulate and cut the arachnoid just lateral to the edge of the tentorium. The temporal lobe opercula can be 'peeled' away from the pia-arachnoid covering the Sylvian fissure and the branches of the middle cerebral artery. By deepening the incision the surgeon dissects through the stem of the temporal lobe into the temporal horn, then proceeding to open the horn up to its full extent.

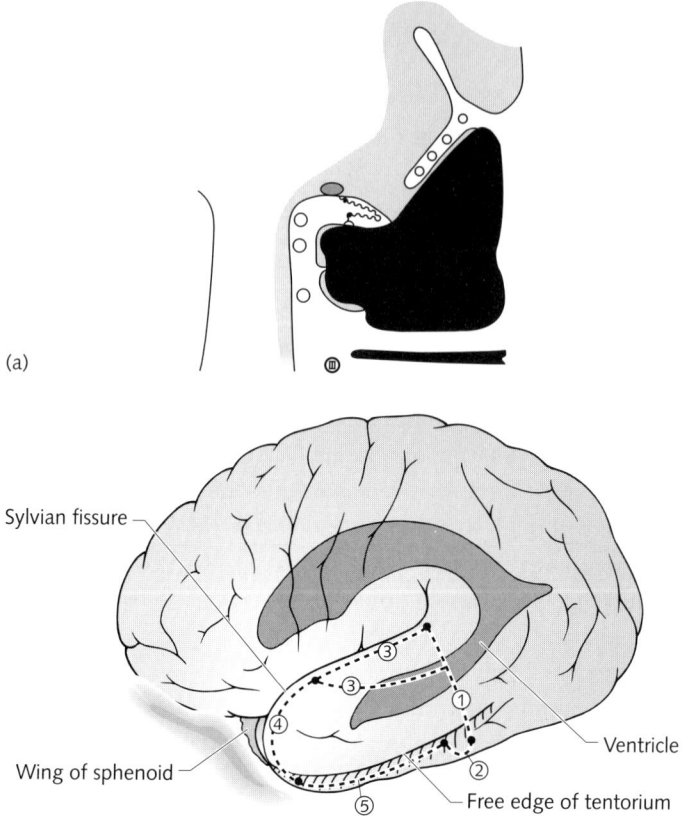

Sylvian fissure

Wing of sphenoid

Ventricle

Free edge of tentorium

Cut ① 6 cm behind temporal pole to enter temporal horn of lateral ventricle
Cut ② Extension inferiorly to free edge of tentorium
Cut ③ Along Sylvian fissure; on the dominant side the posterior 2/3 of the superior temporal gyrus is spread. This incision extends into the temporal horn by working from cut ①
Cut ④ Pia arachnoid cut over temporal pole
Cut ⑤ Pia arachnoid cut just lateral to the free edge of tentorium

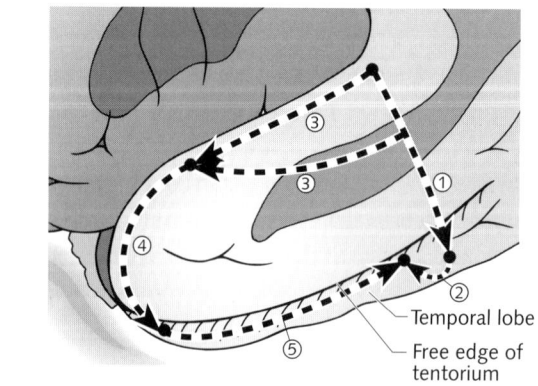

Temporal lobe

Free edge of tentorium

Fig. 46 (a) The *en bloc* temporal lobectomy. (b) Diagram to show order of incisions.

Next the hippocampus is removed by gently sucking through the fimbria, which is exposed by retracting the choroid plexus (Figure 46). At this point the hippocampal sulcus is seen passing forwards and laterally. The vessels of this sulcus need coagulating and cutting, making sure the arachnoid covering the mid-brain is kept intact at all times. The amygdala is grey coloured in contrast to the vivid white hippocampus and sits over the tip of the temporal horn. Most of the amygdala needs to be sucked away. The pathologist will appreciate it if at least the posterior extent is still attached to the specimen if possible. After removal of the specimen the remaining choroid plexus is coagulated to prevent, in effect, an encysted temporal horn. Patients do have a lot of headache for the first post-operative week, presumably due to the large area of exposed dura.

On the dominant side the only difference of technique is to preserve the posterior two-thirds of the superior temporal gyrus. I have performed over 100 temporal lobectomies on the dominant side, under general anaesthesia, without cortical mapping and there has been no lasting post-operative dysphasia using the technique described above.

Amygdalohippocampectomy

Yasargil's sophisticated approach to the temporal horn has two advantages. First, there is no field defect (usually) and secondly, this operation is associated with much less post-operative pain and headache and they make a quicker recovery. The disadvantage is that diffuse temporal lobe pathology cannot be removed. It is ideal for pathology in the region of the hippocampus and amygdala. Once the surgeon has entered the temporal horn the operation proceeds as for removing the amygdala and hippocampus during an *en bloc* temporal lobectomy (Figure 47).

The approach is a pterional flap taken 2 or 3 cm further posteriorly than the standard flap for an aneurysm. The Sylvian fissure is split on the frontal side of the Sylvian vein until it is not possible to proceed further posteriorly because of the branching of the fissure. The main middle cerebral artery and all its major branches are exposed. In doing this the insula with the peri-insular vein is exposed. In my experience the middle cerebral branches are quite variable and sometimes one has to work either side of one of these arteries. An incision is made in the insula and deepened to find the temporal horn. How do you find the temporal horn? I have two guidelines. I advise that when starting to do this operation you expose part of the sphenoid wing. Deepening the incision in the line of the sphenoid wing will bring you to the temporal horn. The other method is to deepen the incision in the same

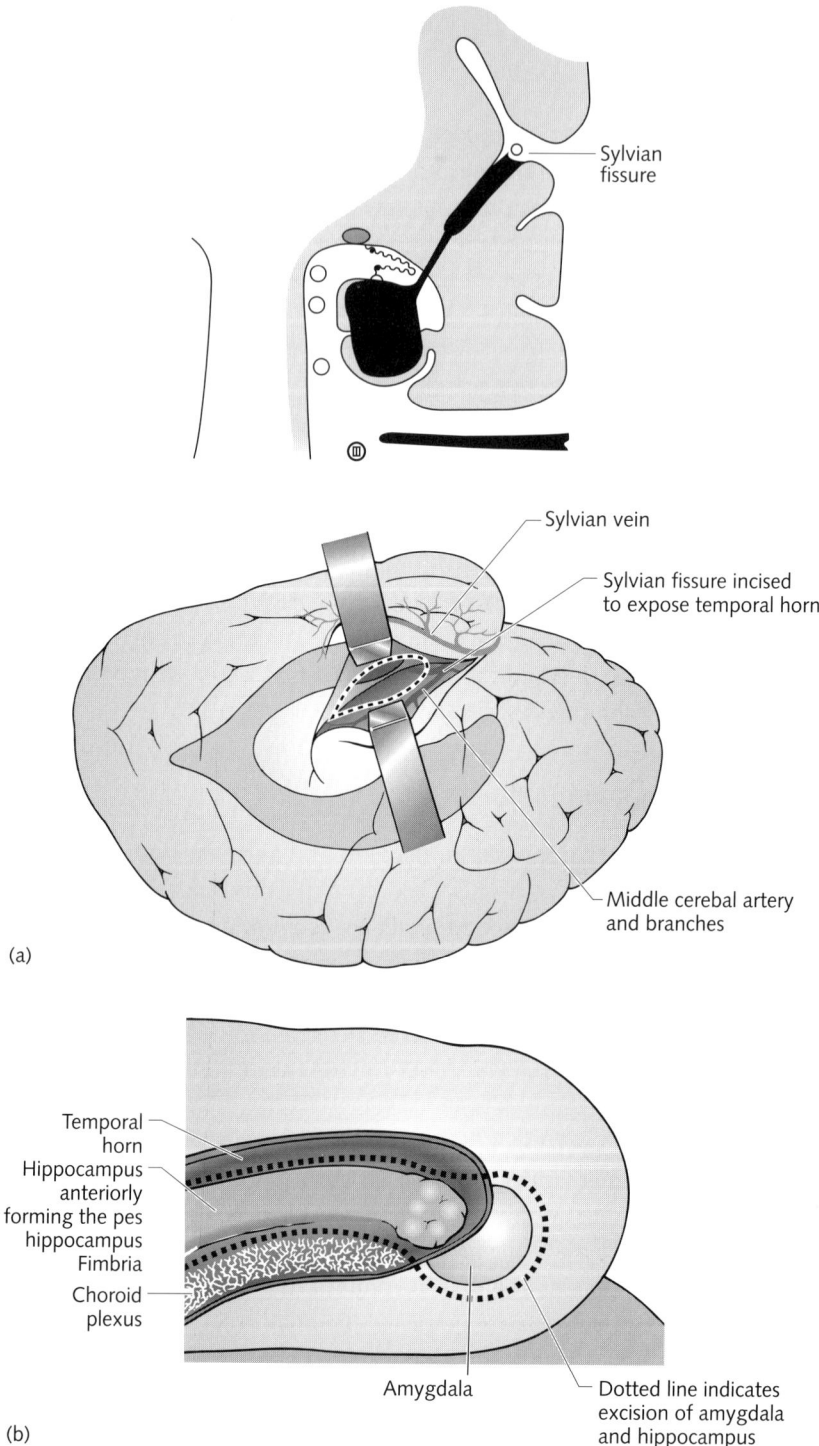

Sylvian
fissure

Sylvian vein

Sylvian fissure incised
to expose temporal horn

Middle cerebal artery
and branches

(a)

Temporal
horn
Hippocampus
anteriorly
forming the pes
hippocampus
Fimbria
Choroid
plexus

Amygdala

Dotted line indicates
excision of amygdala
and hippocampus

(b)

Fig. 47 (a) The Yasargil amygdalohippocampectomy. (b) Diagram to show removal of
hippocampus.

line as the line of the temporal opercula and insula. Look at a coronal view of an MRI scan and you will see what I mean. Once the temporal horn is entered and the incision lengthened to reveal the anterior 3 cm of the hippocampus, the operation proceeds as described earlier. The parahippocampal gyrus is removed as well as the hippocampus and amygdala.

I start lateral to the hippocampus and deepen the incision to the pia mater covering the tentorium (Figure 47). I then extend the incision anteriorly, sucking away by necessity most of the amygdala but preserving what I can. I then retract the choroid plexus to reveal the fimbria and gently suck through this. The hippocampal sulcus needs coagulating and cutting and then finally the posterior cut is made through the hippocampus. As before, the remaining choroid plexus is coagulated.

The amygdalohippocampectomy approach is immensely useful for other pathologies. For instance I have removed a cavernous angioma that had bled four times and had been labelled 'inoperable' because of its situation near to the internal capsule. In fact, using this approach I found the lesion easily, placed in the stem of the temporal lobe extending towards the internal capsule. Once I had dissected to the depths of the Sylvian fissure on the dominant side of the brain, the lesion was, in effect, superficially placed.

Ammon's horn sclerosis: epilepsy surgery

Amygdalohippocampectomy is of course used to treat epilepsy due to Ammon's horn sclerosis, a condition that probably arises at the time of a prolonged (20 minutes +) febrile convulsion in a young (2 years or less), brain. Epilepsy surgery is not immune, like other types of surgery, to fashion. For 25 years I have been convinced that successful surgical treatment of epilepsy must depend on finding and removing focal pathology. In other words this type of surgery is no different to other surgery and has a clearly defined pathological basis but with one qualification. The epilepsy does not arise from the lesion itself but from the cortex surrounding the lesion and so when removing the lesion it is worth taking (if not in an eloquent area of the brain) a centimetre or so of surrounding cortex. If there is a lesion adjacent to the hippocampus and amygdala then my practice is to remove the lesion and the amygdala and hippocampus as these structures seem to play a part in the epileptic process, and the results of surgery are better if these structures are removed as well as the lesion. If the lesion is in, for instance, the posterior part of the temporal lobe then I would remove just the lesion alone.

I have been doing epilepsy surgery since 1972. There is a tendency to make it too complicated. Yes, sometimes it can be difficult to determine if a patient will be helped by surgery and rather than spending huge amounts of money and time on patients whose outcome is uncertain, it would be far better to operate on the straightforward patients who will do well. Epilepsy surgery is under-utilized throughout the world.

To cure a patient of epilepsy is to cure the family and even the community: they are the most grateful of patients. Let me tell you about Jeremy from Manchester. His psychomotor epilepsy (less well called 'complex partial seizures') started at the age of 12; by 16 he was beating up his family and breaking up his home. He had been turned down for surgery by my mentor, Murray Falconer, because of bitemporal independent spikes on the electroencephalogram (EEG). He was referred to me and on the skull X-ray (in 1976 before scans were available) there was a speck of calcification in the right temporal lobe. Because of my belief that finding the pathology was more important than electrical changes I advised a right temporal lobectomy. I found a 1-cm tumour. The post-operative EEG showed all the apparent independent spikes in the opposite temporal lobe had disappeared! He immediately stopped having fits; his behaviour became normal (it always does if you stop the fits, the only exception to this rule being paranoid schizophrenia, which may occur in patients with calcified lesions of the temporal lobe), he passed exams 3 months after the operation, then went to university, became a photographer, got married and thereafter enjoyed a normal life. Do not chase spikes, excise pathology! Moreover, try to operate on young patients so that they can be rehabilitated into society before their schooling is over. They do much better in every way if you can cure the epilepsy when they are still young.

How do you pick patients who are suitable for epilepsy surgery? First take a history. If the fits always start in the same way then you should be encouraged as it suggests a constant focal origin. It does not matter how the fits develop, but if the fit always starts in the same way, particularly if of a focal nature then go further. This means do an MRI scan and measure hippocampal volumes. You must then do an EEG; sphenoidal electrodes with the patient asleep will provide an enormous amount of information in patients with temporal lobe epilepsy and will allow confirmation that the structural scan changes relate to the epileptic activity. It is remarkable how often benign gliomas/hamartomas cause epilepsy to start around the age of 12, although these lesions have probably been present since birth. Also, a helpful lateralizing sign is the transient weakness down the contralateral side one sees after a febrile convulsion; this information can only be obtained from the parents or relatives, of course. I suspect the hemiplegia, epilepsy syndrome that so often occurs aged 1 or 2 after febrile illness and which may lead to a hemispherectomy of a profoundly damaged hemisphere, may be an extension of this transient hemiplegia seen after a febrile convulsion.

In summary, 80% of surgically treated patients have pathology in the temporal lobe and 80% of these patients can be assessed by four simple approaches: a careful history and examination, an MRI scan, simple non-invasive EEG studies and a carotid amytal test (to assess speech and memory). Operate on young patients for the best overall results. The KISS principle again!

Hemispherectomy

This is still the best operation for stopping epilepsy. The reference at the end of this book (Adams, in press) is a useful starting point for those interested in this operation. The surgery itself is not difficult and will not be discussed further here.

Aneurysm surgery

Aneurysm surgery is well established, and I have no intention of discussing routine aneurysm surgery. I would stress a few aspects that I feel are not widely known or perhaps have been forgotten. Through experience, at times rather bitter experience, I have learned to avoid not only operations but also angiography between the fourth and eighth day after the bleed. Days six/seven are the most frequent time for 'vasospasm' or more correctly non-haemorrhagic neurological deterioration associated with a narrow lumen of two or more major vessels on angiography. There has been prolonged, even acrimonious discussion about whether vasospasm is associated with clinical deterioration. The answer I believe is that vasospasm affecting one vessel is not usually associated with clinical deterioration but if two or more vessels (i.e. internal carotid artery or the main middle cerebral or anterior cerebral artery) are affected then inevitably there is clinical deterioration. I have learned that one must not only time surgery but also angiography and to avoid the fourth to the eighth days. If the brain is suffering from ischaemia, to replace a column of blood by a column of dye may just be sufficient to cause clinical deterioration.

I think it is often forgotten that the following factors affect the outcome and should, if present, persuade the surgeon to consider delayed surgery (i.e. 10 days or more after the bleed) rather than early surgery in the first 72 hours. These factors are firstly the age of the patient (over 50), secondly, hypertension especially if untreated and thirdly, the presence of a neurological deficit. I have seen patients in grade 3 or 4, even grade 5, make remarkable recoveries if left alone and the surgeon stays his or her hand. Much better functional recoveries are made by waiting and operating when the patient has improved. There is a fashion for early surgery, which may indeed prevent early rebleeding but it is undoubtedly much more difficult to carry out. I am quite prepared to admit this even though I have operated on more than 1000 patients with aneurysms. No randomized trial has shown that early surgery produces better management mortality and morbidity rates compared with delayed surgery at 10 days after the bleed. The problem is that the literature contains papers published by surgeons who perhaps specialize in aneurysm surgery and their results are good—or they would not publish them! I suspect the results of early surgery practised by non-publishing and less experienced surgeons may be very different!

Vasospasm

Vasospasm is a most remarkable phenomenon. I once waited 4 weeks before operating on a patient with an anterior communicating artery aneurysm who had developed vasospasm. When I eventually operated he died postoperatively due to intense vasospasm. At post-mortem the aneurysm that bled was in fact a vertebro-basilar aneurysm undiagnosed, for in those days routine vertebral angiography (by direct puncture of a vertebral artery) was not carried out. The CSF taken at post-mortem was injected by a colleague in London, into a baboon and this induced severe vasospasm of the baboon's blood vessels. Thus, operating on the wrong aneurysm but releasing a further dose of blood into the 'primed' system was sufficient to induce fatal vasospasm by a substance that seems transmitted in the CSF and to only develop 3 or so days after the initial bleed. I wish I was more convinced that calcium blockers prevented or relieved vasospasm but I am not. I use them with considerable reluctance and suspect no one will use them in 5 years' time.

There is one further general aspect of aneurysmal subarachnoid haemorrhage that has perhaps received less attention than it deserves. After a bleed the adrenaline and noradrenaline blood levels increase to the sort of levels seen with a phaeochromocytoma. Why this happens I do not know. What effect this has I am not sure but I personally favour putting my patients on beta-blocking agents, which certainly seem to smooth out the hypertensive swings these patients may sometimes show.

Retinal haemorrhages of course may be seen. I always imagined they occurred at the time of the release of blood into the intracranial cavity producing a sudden rise of intracranial pressure. I once was examining a patient's fundi 3 hours or so after the bleed and saw appearing at that moment retinal haemorrhages bursting out in various directions. I do not have an explanation; it is an observation.

Aneurysms of the anterior circle of Willis: general principles

I had not intended to discuss general principles and the approach to aneurysms of the internal carotid artery, middle cerebral and anterior communicating arteries. However, I recently appeared as an expert witness in a court of law when three experienced consultant neurosurgeons stated they approached posterior communicating artery aneurysms by retracting the orbital surface of the frontal lobe while simultaneously retracting the temporal lobe. Having practised all my professional life, splitting the Sylvian fissure in order to expose the internal carotid artery and its branches with minimal retraction of the frontal lobe and without recourse to retracting the temporal lobe, I had imagined that every other neurosurgeon did the same. Clearly this is not the case. Retractors should be avoided if at all possible; not only do they damage the brain but they increase the likelihood of rupture of the aneurysm. Of course two retractors are much more likely to rupture the aneurysm when applied simultaneously to the frontal and temporal lobes and retraction applied in different directions. The key to approaching aneurysms of the anterior circle of Willis is to split the Sylvian fissure and this technique has already been discussed. It is important to cut the arachnoid using sharp dissection (rather than tear it) and to routinely extend the arachnoid dissection over the optic nerve to the midline. By doing this the frontal lobe will fall away from the temporal lobe and the circle of Willis, with little or no retraction of the frontal lobe. Just occasionally the temporal lobe has to be 'retained' in its normal position but retraction is quite unnecessary and indeed dangerous.

I position the patient with the malar eminence on the side of the lesion uppermost. It is, of course, necessary to carry out a pterional bone flap taken low down onto the floor of the anterior cranial fossa. When splitting the Sylvian fissure one has to direct the microscope laterally to see 'under' the temporal opercula. If one is operating on an anterior communicating artery aneurysm one eventually moves the microscope nearly 180° so that it becomes directed medially when dissecting the neck of the anterior communicating artery aneurysm. It pays to split the fissure slowly to allow CSF to escape which aids the falling away of the frontal lobe. I find mannitol or a diuretic useful as well. I do not put in a lumbar drain, preferring to maintain the subarachnoid space, which aids finding the correct pial planes when splitting the fissure. If the brain is very tight it usually means there is a marked communicating hydrocephalus, and a ventricular drain can make all the difference. The third point of a 2.5 cm equilateral triangle, one side being along the most proximally exposed part of the Sylvian fissure with the apex or third point lying over the frontal lobe, is the point to insert a ventricular needle at right angles to the brain. I then tunnel a ventricular catheter through the scalp with an open barrel of a syringe containing Ringers solution, attached to the end of the catheter. Passing the other end of the catheter into the brain with the syringe elevated will indicate entry into the ventricle when the level of the fluid falls in the syringe barrel.

When approaching the aneurysm one must obtain proximal control as soon as possible, so that a temporary clip can be applied should the aneurysm rupture. If one is operating on a middle cerebral artery aneurysm one must very cautiously split the fissure to allow one to get to the internal carotid and main middle cerebral arteries and hence obtain proximal control, before dissecting more deeply in the fissure. Likewise for an anterior communicating artery aneurysm one must find both anterior cerebral arteries (usually by dissecting deep to the aneurysm just above the optic chiasm) before approaching the aneurysm sac. After proximal control has been obtained one must then dissect out all the adjacent vessels, again avoiding the neck of the aneurysm to the last possible moment. All the time the surgeon must plan what to do should the aneurysm rupture. The surgeon must have in his or her mind's eye what structures the sac of the aneurysm is attached to and avoid retraction, which will cause tension on the sac. If necessary, dissect through the pia to release the sac of the aneurysm if it is adherent or invaginated into the brain. This will allow safer retraction but will also allow safer dissection by having a layer of pia between you and the aneurysm sac. This is a worthwhile manoeuvre if the aneurysm is very thin walled.

It is remarkable how with the operating microscope one can dissect vessels away from the aneurysm to define the neck. I find careful bipolar coagulation helpful by slightly thickening the aneurysm wall while dissecting vessels away from the aneurysm sac. Personally I do not like using dissectors around the neck but prefer to use fine bipolar forceps so I can use coagulation in the way just described. I also find dissectors go through the neck rather too easily for my liking! I do not often use hypotension these days but I have no hesitation in using temporary clips electively to dissect around the aneurysm neck. One can apply the clip for 5 minutes then release the clip to allow the blood to recirculate. This is particularly useful when drilling off the anterior clinoid process adjacent to aneurysm; then of course one must obtain proximal control of the internal carotid artery in the neck.

If the aneurysm ruptures, apply the sucker to the hole and by angling the sucker one can often stop the bleeding and allow the clip to be quickly applied to the neck. If one has proximal control and immediate clipping of the neck is not possible then apply a temporary clip (or clips), complete the neck dissection and then clip the neck of the aneurysm. I still think thiopentone is a useful adjunct when temporary clips are used. I ask to be told each minute that passes, but I have had temporary clips on for 20 minutes without harm to the patient. It obviously depends on the degree of co-lateral circulation but clearly one keeps temporary clips on for the least possible time. Usually it is not necessary to apply temporary clips for more than 5 minutes.

If the neck of the aneurysm is wide or if the sac is worryingly tense (possibly causing the clip to cut through the neck of the aneurysm or for the clip to slide off the neck onto the artery) then it is best to apply temporary clips on the artery before clipping the neck of the aneurysm. The measures needed for clipping a giant aneurysm are discussed in a later section. Almost invariably I use a straight clip for the neck because the 1–2-cm exposure does not allow more than a straight clip. Occasionally, difficult internal carotid artery aneurysms need angled clips, applied in series, but these occasions are rare. Posterior communicating artery aneurysms can be easy, but they can also be very difficult, if for instance the sac is hiding under the tentorial edge. I find it helpful to apply a straight clip with my left hand for a left posterior communicating aneurysm; the clip goes on at a better angle and I do not usually worry about trying to preserve the posterior communicating artery itself. I have never regretted my lack of worry in this respect.

If the clip fails to entirely occlude the aneurysm sac, wrap wisps of cotton wool around the proximal sac and artery. These induce a fibrotic reaction and rather surprisingly I have no record of any rebleeding or 'blowing out' of the remaining aneurysm sac in these circumstances, nor have I seen a harmful granuloma develop using cotton wool in this way.

The essence of aneurysm surgery is to creep to the neck of the aneurysm with minimal brain retraction. First obtain proximal control, then dissect the vessels and only finally define the neck of the aneurysm immediately prior to clipping it. I have included at the back of this book reference to Gazi Yasargil's superbly illustrated volumes on aneurysm surgery. These are unlikely to be surpassed as endovascular therapists will treat increasing numbers of these aneurysms in the future.

Basilar bifurcation aneurysms

Despite the advent of endovascular treatment of aneurysms, there are still occasions when a surgeon needs to clip a basilar bifurcation aneurysm. The crucial thing is to preserve the perforating arteries arising from the first part of the posterior cerebral arteries (P1 segment) either side of the neck of the aneurysm. I have tried all the various ways to operate on these aneurysms and I have no doubt that the best way is an antero-lateral approach, removing the tip of the temporal lobe to expose the third nerve then the posterior communicating artery. This can be traced back to the posterior cerebral artery as it winds around the mid-brain. This vessel is seen routinely through the arachnoid during a temporal lobectomy or amygdalohippocampectomy. Removing the tip (2–3 cm) of the temporal lobe is less traumatic than elevating it and the exposure is far better than the pterional approach opening Lillequist's membrane. The antero-lateral approach allows these all-important P1 perforators to be identified on both sides of the neck of the aneurysm. It also allows a temporary clip to be put on the basilar trunk, which the 'skull base' approach removing the zygomatic arch does not so easily allow. If need be, further exposure can be obtained by placing a suture through the edge of the tentorium to retract it laterally thus improving the inferior exposure. This is sometimes necessary for a low-lying basilar bifurcation aneurysm or to place a temporary clip on the basilar artery. Once I had to carry out an emergency craniotomy for a basilar bifurcation aneurysm when an endovascular coil had ruptured the aneurysm but the coil itself had also herniated into the basilar artery (Figure 48). Using this approach I was able to place a temporary clip on the basilar artery, remove the coil through the fundus of the aneurysm then clip the aneurysm neck. The patient made a very good recovery.

Posterior inferior cerebellar artery aneurysms

I have no doubt that the easiest way to approach a posterior inferior cerebellar artery (PICA) aneurysm is a midline approach, preferably with the patient in a sitting position. The secret is to retract the cerebellar tonsil superiorly and in this way one can identify the PICA medially and the verte-

---

Fig. 48 (a) Angiogram showing basilar bifurcation aneurysm (that had bled). (b) Endovascular coil had penetrated the aneurysm sac but of more importance a coil loop has herniated into the basilar artery, threatening to cause a thrombosis. (*Continued*)

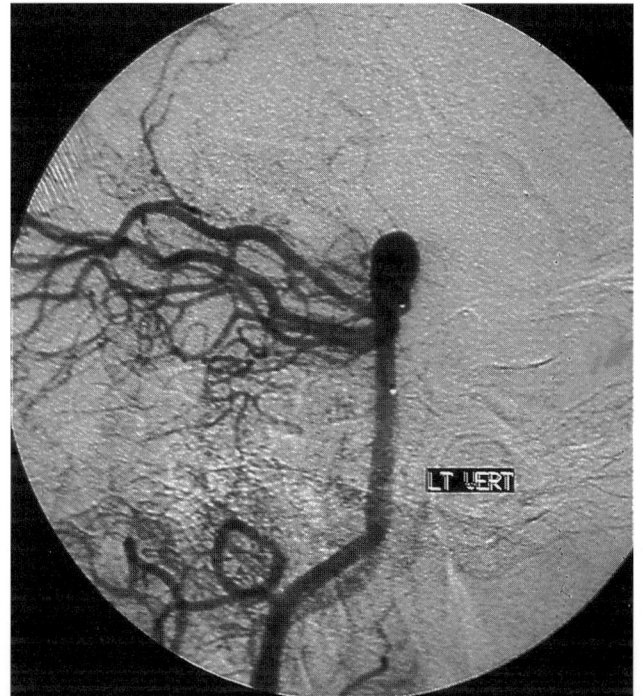

(a)

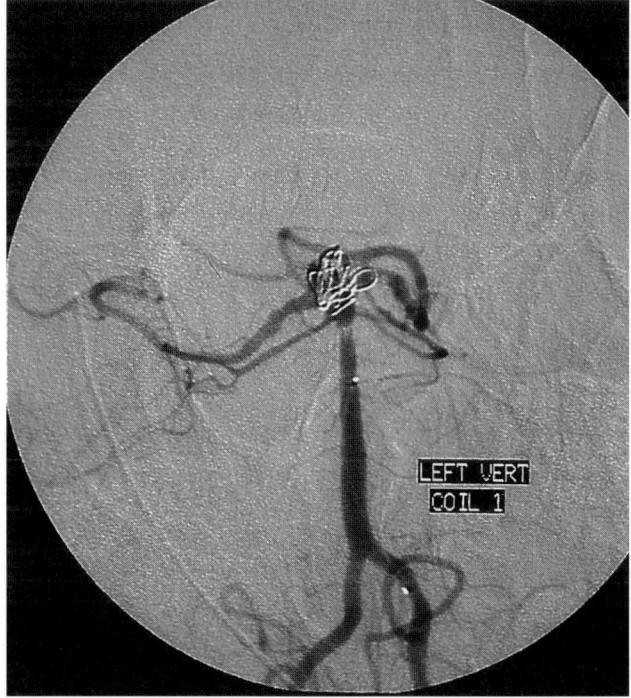

(b)

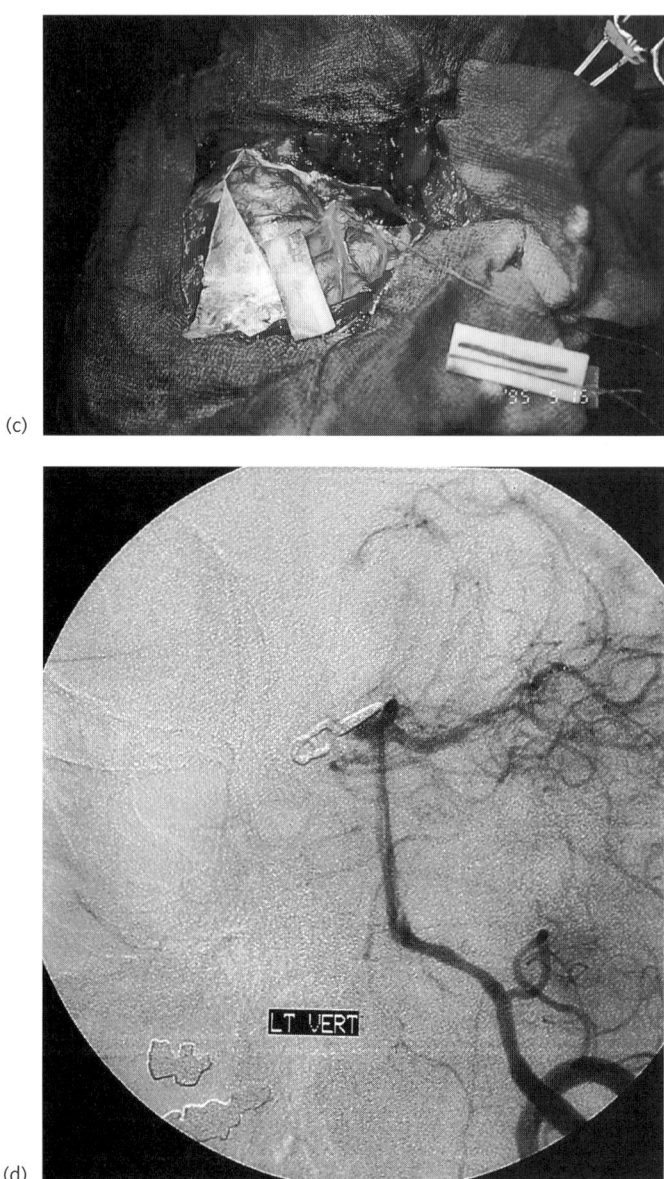

(c)

(d)

Fig. 48 (*Continued*) (c) Emergency surgery; the tip of the temporal lobe and inferior temporal gyrus was excised to allow access to the basilar artery and its branches. A temporary clip was placed on the basilar artery, the coil removed through the fundus of the aneurysm, which was then clipped. (d) Post-operative angiogram. The patient made a complete recovery.

bral artery laterally. By tracing these two vessels superiorly by gradually increasing the retraction of the cerebellar tonsil, the surgeon reaches the origin of the PICA from the vertebral artery and finds the aneurysm nestling between the two. A lateral approach is much more difficult, but using this midline approach and retracting the tonsil upwards has allowed me to clip these aneurysms without undue difficulty. Try it! This 'inferior' approach moreover allows you early proximal control of the vertebral artery and also allows you to apply the clip along the line of the vertebral artery. It makes this operation easy and certainly conforms to the KISS principle! My impression is that these aneurysms are associated with a higher than usual incidence of symptomatic communicating hydrocephalus.

Giant basilar trunk aneurysms

My operative mortality for this group is 100%, I regret to say. The efforts of the endovascular experts have not been much better because their problem and my problem have been the same. When the aneurysm sac thromboses (I too have tried snares around the vertebral artery occluding the artery post-operatively under X-ray control) the perforating arteries arising from the adjacent basilar trunk have become occluded by the propagating thrombus. My future strategy will probably rely on occlusion of the more proximal vertebral artery in the neck, in an effort to reduce the inflow pressure into the aneurysm. These are thoroughly unpleasant lesions and we do not have a good answer to them yet.

Ophthalmic aneurysms

These are not as difficult as they are reputed to be. One needs proximal control and I obtain this by exposing the internal carotid artery in the neck. One also needs curiously angled aneurysm clips because the neck is often rather wide. It is necessary to expose the internal carotid artery as it emerges from the cavernous sinus because the neck of the aneurysm arises here. Often cutting the dural component of the optic foramen is sufficient to expose the ophthalmic artery and define the neck of the aneurysm, but if not, then the anterior clinoid process needs to be drilled away. If in doubt, drill off the anterior clinoid process as it makes the placement of a clip much easier and safer.

Giant aneurysms

To place a clip on a giant aneurysm you often need to do two things. First, empty the aneurysm sac of blood by putting temporary clips on the relevant artery and then puncturing the fundus with a needle and applying a sucker to the hole, which usually has the effect of collapsing the sac down and allowing clips to be applied. One word of advice is to make sure your needle puncture is well distal towards the fundus. When the sac collapses a more proximally made puncture can migrate rather too close to the neck of the aneurysm for comfort. The second thing to be done is to be sure your clip is placed precisely at the neck of the aneurysm. If placed slightly too distally blood in the remaining neck of the giant aneurysm will 'pump' the clip either off the aneurysm or at least force the blades of the clip open. If one places the clip exactly at the neck flush with the line of the artery then this does not happen. A group of smaller clips in series, the first one being fenestrated, often allows more forcible neck occlusion than using a longer bladed aneurysm clip. In the late 1970s I used profound hypothermia and cardiopulmonary bypass to operate on a series of giant aneurysms. The results were reasonable (no mortality in five cases) but I felt the difficulties and complexity outweighed the advantages. The KISS principle was violated!

Pericallosal aneurysms

Use a parasagittal flap; do not try to find the aneurysm or the pericallosal arteries until you have found the corpus callosum. This is white and avascular. If you do not find this first you will get lost! Having found it you will then know for sure which arteries are the pericallosal arteries and which are the calloso-marginal arteries. Trace these proximally and you will (usually) find the aneurysm at the junction of the pericallosal and callosal marginal arteries. From there on, these are usually easy.

Pituitary surgery

Trans-sphenoidal surgery is well established. It requires two things: first the surgeon, whether he or she approaches sublabially or trans-nasally, must find the midline and stick to it, and secondly, the tumour must not be a hard one! The midline is easily found when the operation is the first one. It may be extremely difficult to find when operating for a recurrent tumour. Although I have a very large experience of this type of surgery I have abandoned the operation on two occasions because of a complete inability to find the midline, coupled with an inability to know where the internal carotid arteries were. In these circumstances there is the trans-cranial option and difficult as it is to abandon any operation, I felt it is safer to do so in these circumstances. On one occasion, having abandoned the operation, I came back again trans-sphenoidally another day, finding the midline and completing the operation without undue difficulty.

I learned my lesson concerning hard pituitary tumours early in my experience. Fortunately hard pituitary tumours are rare. (Hard lesions may also be due to hypophysitis or metastases in the pituitary gland.) I attempted to do too much; the tumour became swollen and would not of course descend into the cavity I had tried to create. Post-operatively the patient deteriorated and I had to perform an emergency craniotomy but I regret the patient was left intellectually impaired. Size is not a contra-indication to the trans-sphenoidal approach but a hard tumour certainly is. When I find a hard tumour I do nothing except take a biopsy and pack the sphenoid sinus. The latter may seem strange at the time with a large hard tumour between you and the CSF but if you do not do this you will regret it when you carry out a trans-frontal craniotomy and find a patent anterior wall of the pituitary fossa leading into the sphenoid sinus.

Once I tried biopsying a cavernous sinus meningioma by this approach and for reasons I do not entirely understand, this was not successful. The angle of approach, although tempting on the MRI scan, proved much more difficult to achieve in practice, and I will not try this again.

Before the advent of scans, on two occasions I came across an intrasellar aneurysm. Fortunately on both occasions the tense, pulsating mass was clearly an aneurysm and the operation was terminated without even 'needling' the tumour. I don't advocate needling in these circumstances. An awful lot of blood can come out of a needled aneurysm, which can be extremely difficult to control. If in doubt come out and do an angiogram. If you are wrong and it is not an aneurysm no harm will have been done.

My one operative death was an experience I would not wish to repeat. I had reached no further than the sphenoid sinus when the blood pressure rose over a few seconds to over 250 mm systolic. The patient started bleeding ferociously from more than one area and I could only control the bleeding by packing. She had an undiagnosed phaeochromocytoma and died from intracranial haemorrhage. I never saw the pituitary tumour. Since then we have had a high index of suspicion and carry out a 24-hour urinary collection looking for evidence of phaeochromocytoma if there is any possibility of such a lesion being present. Patients on medical treatment for Parkinson's disease can cause similar urinary changes to a phaeochromocytoma, so do not be confused in this situation.

There are two other occasions, fortunately much less serious, when bleeding may be a problem. The first is operating on a small tumour, usually for Cushing's syndrome. With these small pituitary tumours, the circular venous sinus has not been obliterated by tumour compression and however assiduous the surgeon has been in coagulating the dura prior to incising it, there may be ferocious venous bleeding. Although I try to control this with Surgicel I am not usually successful and I find it best to continue the operation using a large sucker to control the bleeding and then to rapidly find and remove the tumour. Once the tumour is out, this bleeding, like all venous bleeding quickly stops with Surgicel, pressure and patience. One must warn the anaesthetist of this bleeding because one can exsanguinate a patient very quickly in these circumstances. The only group of patients undergoing trans-sphenoidal surgery that I cross-match for blood are the patients with Cushing's syndrome.

The other circumstance where bleeding may be a problem is removing a large tumour that has invaded the clivus. After the tumour removal there is a large area of bleeding cancellous bone. As long as no CSF has been seen I find it useful in these circumstances to leave a suction drain in the cavity and bring it down adjacent to the nasal septum, bringing it out through the incision in the mucosa of the upper lip. It stays for 24 hours and since using this I have not had to remove a post-operative haematoma (Figure 49).

Normal anterior lobe, yellow and firm is quite different from tumour, which is pale, usually soft, and 'flaky' rather like Campbell's condensed mushroom soup. Posterior pituitary tissue looks like brain, which of course it is! Pathologists seem to have more difficulty than surgeons in identifying tumour from normal tissue. Some 30% of patients with Cushing's syndrome that I cure (i.e. I must have removed something pathological!) have a histological report stating 'normal pituitary tissue'. Initially my reaction was one of paranoia but nowadays I believe it raises an interesting question about why pathologists have difficulty in recognizing the difference between normal pituitary and tumour. Any reasonably experienced pituitary surgeon knows which is 'obvious' tumour; it may be more difficult when the tumour merges with the normal, however.

It is rare to damage normal pituitary function because in my experience the normal pituitary tissue is usually pushed superiorly (Figure 50). Often the posterior lobe can be recognized on the pre-operative MRI scan as a

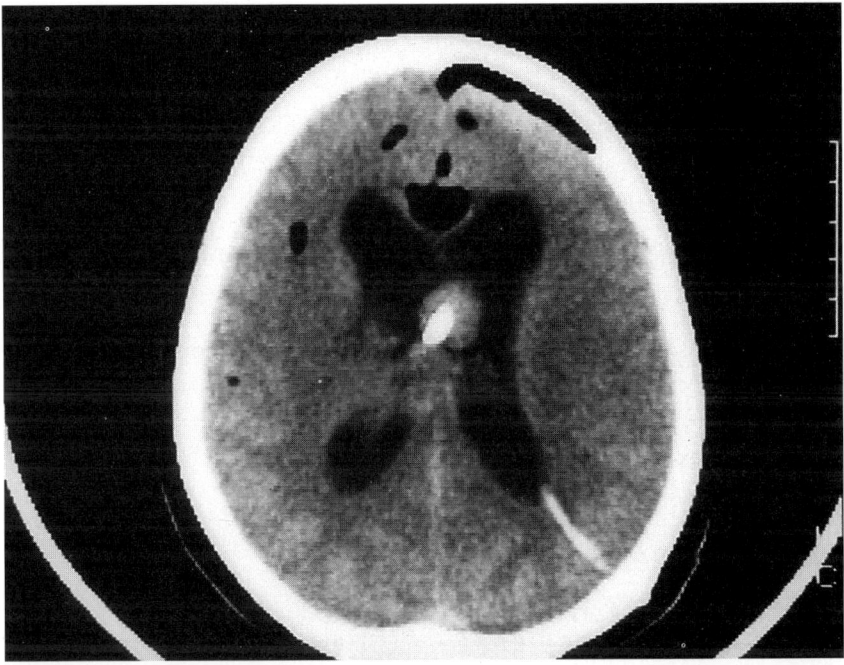

Fig. 49 Post-operative CT scan following trans-sphenoidal removal of a large pituitary tumour. If there is no CSF leakage, I have found it useful to insert a drain into the cavity (as shown). Bring the drain out through the nasal cavity and sublabial incision, suturing it to the cheek. I only use this when there is a large operative cavity especially with exposed bleeding cancellous bone (of the clivus) and when I am fearful of a post-operative haematoma.

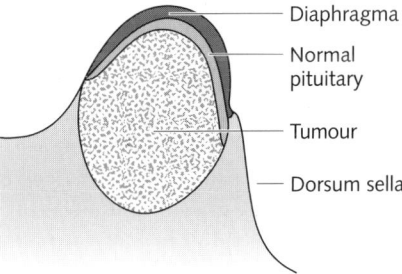

Diaphragma

Normal
pituitary

Tumour

Dorsum sella

Fig. 50 Diagram to show why pituitary function is usually preserved after trans-sphenoidal surgery and usually destroyed after trans-cranial surgery.

high-density nodule. If I see CSF I always use fascia lata to reinforce the diaphragma and fill the pituitary fossa with fat. I also find it useful to obliterate the sphenoid sinus, thus removing the adjacent 'dead space'. This additional measure reduces the post-operative CSF leakage rate considerably. If no CSF is seen then Surgicel is sufficient for packing the pituitary fossa. Do not put too much Surgicel in as it swells and may itself cause chiasmal compression. I always give my patients a 5-day course of antibiotics and this reduces the incidence of meningitis to a very low level.

One last comment concerning the difficulty in finding the midline; if you cannot see your sucker exactly against the pituitary fossa on the X-ray monitor then it is not applied to the fossa and you are to one side of the midline. Usually the fossa is the most posteriorly placed structure in the sphenoid sinus. If, when reoperating on a pituitary tumour, you cannot find the midline or the pituitary fossa, I repeat my advice to abandon the operation rather than risk damage to a carotid artery.

Headache: salt-losing syndrome

Before leaving the pituitary fossa and its contents it is worth mentioning some potential medical problems. The most frightening is 'salt-losing syndrome'. This may come on a week or two after the operation and after the patient has gone home. The patient develops a headache: think of nasal sinus haematoma (common), CSF leak (fairly common), meningitis (rare but do a lumbar puncture; the post-operative antibiotics may mask meningitis), pituitary abscess (write it up if you diagnose and treat it; do an MRI scan and look for a ring shadow in the pituitary fossa) and finally do the electrolytes; you may find a low sodium. Salt-losing syndrome is potentially lethal and it does exist. I have had one patient with it and she survived. Put in a central venous line to decide if the low sodium is due to water over-load or salt wasting. The management of this condition is debated. We resuscitated our patient with a rapid infusion of fluids and salt and then cautiously fluid restricted her. Until this condition is better understood the management will be a matter of trying to treat the fluid and electrolyte abnormalities rather empirically.

Diabetes insipidus

We avoid diuretics and mannitol during pituitary surgery. We restrict fluids to 2 litres a day for 48 hours post-operatively. A post-operative diuresis is normal, especially in patients with acromegaly. But measure the urinary output; if this is more than 200 ml/hour for 3 hours then do the plasma and urine osmolality. If the former is more (and the latter less) than 295 mosmol/kg then give desmopressin. Repeat the osmolalities in 24 hours or longer depending on the urinary output.

As a surgeon I have always been confused that 20 mg of cortisone by mouth is equivalent to 100 mg given intramuscularly or intravenously, but it is so, and there we are.

The 'secondary' empty sella causing optic nerve or chiasmal damage

Do you believe this? I don't. Let me explain. It used to be stated that the herniated optic nerves and chiasm into the now empty pituitary fossa following removal of a pituitary tumour, can be damaged and hence produce visual impairment. Perhaps as Guiot states it can happen acutely, but I have never seen it and I marvel why I have not, when one rapidly removes a large pituitary tumour and the previously stretched and elevated diaphragma now lies on the floor of the pituitary fossa. I analysed the reported cases in the literature and found the visual failure came on about a year later, the visual loss was often sudden and unilateral. These are characteristics of optic radiation damage and all the reported patients had had radiotherapy in larger doses than normal. I believe the 'secondary empty sella syndrome' is due to radiotherapy damage to the optic nerve and chiasm. So don't bother to do 'chiasmopexy' operations to elevate the fallen chiasm!

Acoustic neuromas

Harvey Cushing dubbed this 'the gloomy corner of neurosurgery'. These days it is less gloomy but a large vascular acoustic neuroma is one of the greatest challenges for a neurosurgeon. There are two particular areas of neurosurgical frustration. First, the patient always appears relatively well pre-operatively and the best a surgeon can achieve is to maintain that pre-operative state. Secondly, the neurosurgeon can always do better. If you are pleased your patient has an intact and working facial nerve post-operatively what about next time preserving the hearing?!

I have tried all ways of approaching these tumours and feel the retrosigmoid, suboccipital approach is the best. This allows hearing preservation. The blood supply to these tumours is from the dura around the internal auditory meatus as well as from the intracranial vessels, mainly the anterior inferior cerebellar artery. Pre-operative embolization is impossible but I find hypotension during the surgery to be especially helpful and recommend it particularly when trying to dissect tumour away from the brain stem and cranial nerves. The anterior inferior cerebellar artery loops onto the tumour and then back to the brain stem, and the importance of preserving this vessel is well known.

Maintaining a plane when dissecting the tumour is essential. It is helpful to have an understanding of how the arachnoid becomes distributed around the tumour (Figures 51 and 52). Soft acoustic neuromas may be in one way more difficult to dissect from the brain stem because of similar consistencies, but soft tumours damage the surroundings less and often the facial nerve is found to be a nice discrete bundle in these circumstances. The only place where the tumour is attached to the brain stem is at the point of attachment of the eighth nerve. One needs immense patience to 'maintain the correct plane'. If bleeding occurs whilst dissecting you have probably lost the correct plane—go somewhere else and find it and then work your way around to where you were before.

There are several signposts to the facial nerve medially. The first is the flocculus of the cerebellum. When this is retracted one sees a vein, the vein of the lateral recess which joins with the petrosal vein. Next, one sees the eighth nerve, especially the cochlear nerve curling around the lower pole of the tumour. Just below this is the choroid plexus emerging from the foramen of Luschka and it is here one picks up the vagal and glossopharyngeal nerves. Just above this point, usually in the vicinity of the anterior inferior cerebellar artery, is the facial nerve where it emerges rather gradually from the brain stem (Figure 52(b)).

The first thing to do when one exposes an acoustic neuroma is to let off CSF by opening a cistern, usually around the vagal group of nerves. If the tumour is large then a lumbar puncture drain may be useful to allow CSF to be released before opening the dura. My general approach to the removal of an acoustic neuroma is first to dissect around the cerebellum and brain stem side of the tumour to try to find the medial end of the facial nerve before the tissue plane has been stained with blood. If the tumour is large this is not possible until some debulking has been done. It is very helpful to have a motorized table to allow the tumour to be moved around the microscope rather than vice versa. I have stopped using the ultrasonic aspirator for debulking the tumour and now use bipolar coagulation or, if the tumour is very soft, suction. After this phase I move to drill off the back of the internal auditory meatus while the bleeding from the tumour cavity subsides. There are two tips concerning the meatus. First, be beware of the occasional jugular bulb that overlies the meatus. This can cause impressive venous bleeding if drilled into. Secondly, do not be tempted to drill too little of the meatus. One can

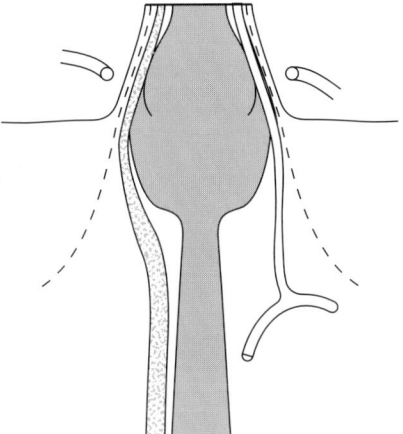

(a)

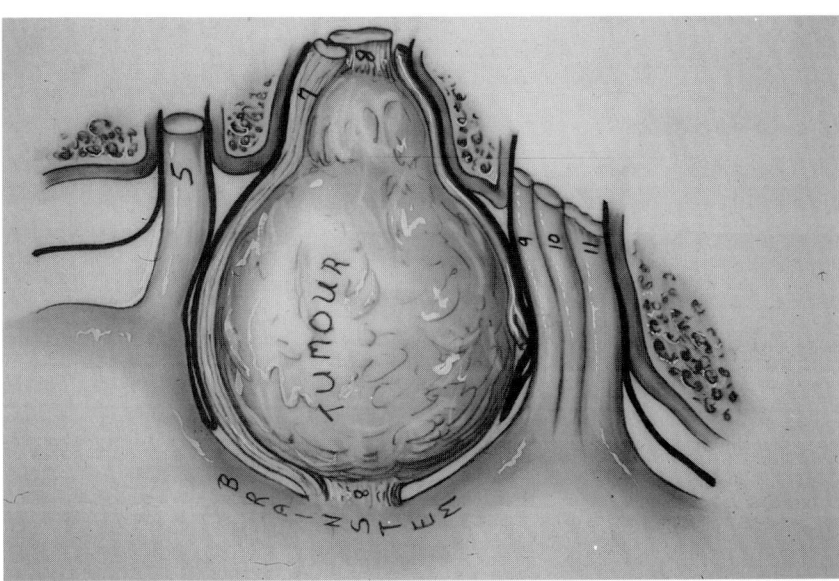

(b)

Fig. 51 (a,b) The distribution of arachnoid around the acoustic neuroma is crucial to the removal of the tumour. Look at the normal distribution of the arachnoid, it is a funnel around the seventh and eighth nerves entering the IAM. When the tumour arises just medial to the meatus it invaginates itself into the arachnoid as shown diagrammatically. When it arises more medially it does not have an arachnoid layer around it and it becomes much more difficult to remove, especially if it is cystic (see Figure 13, pp. 18–19).

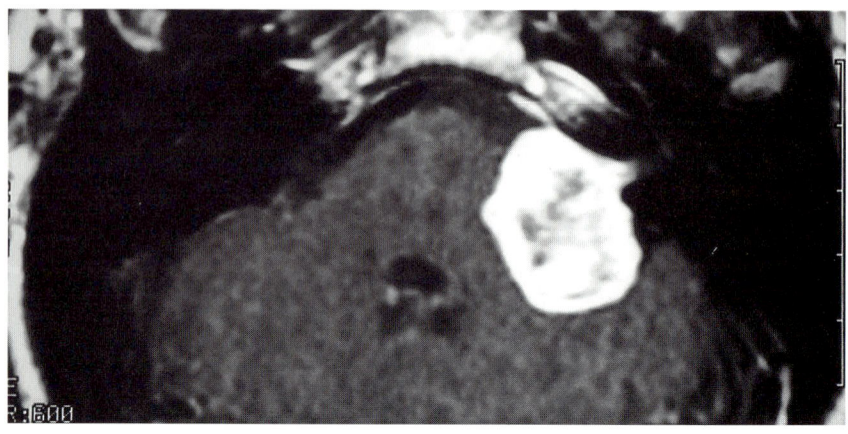

(a)

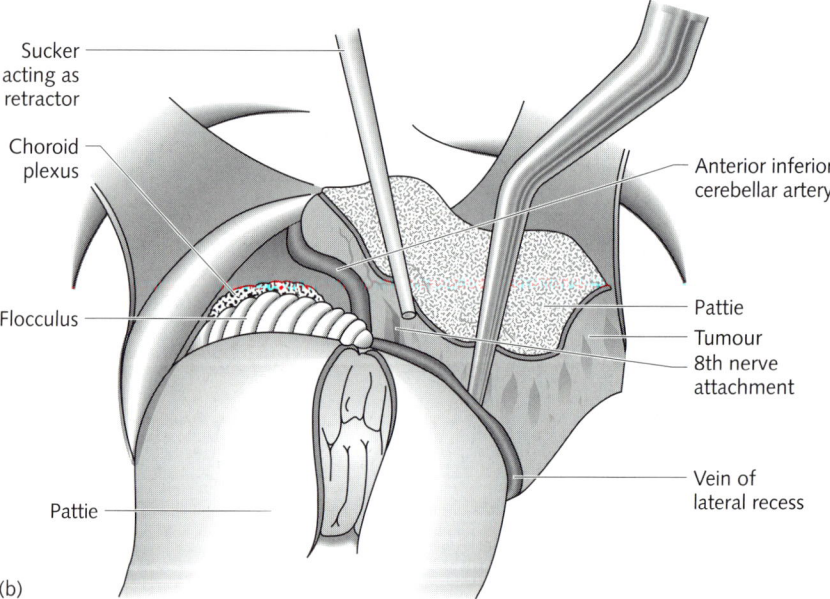

Sucker
acting as
retractor

Choroid
plexus

Anterior inferior
cerebellar artery

Flocculus

Pattie

Tumour

8th nerve
attachment

Vein of
lateral recess

Pattie

(b)

Fig. 52 (a) MRI scan of an acoustic neuroma. One can see the subarachnoid space around part of the tumour. (b) Diagram to show the 'signposts' to the medial end of the seventh nerve: first the flocculus, then the vein of the lateral recess, next the choroid plexus, and finally the eighth nerve and anterior inferior cerebellar artery. (*Continued*)

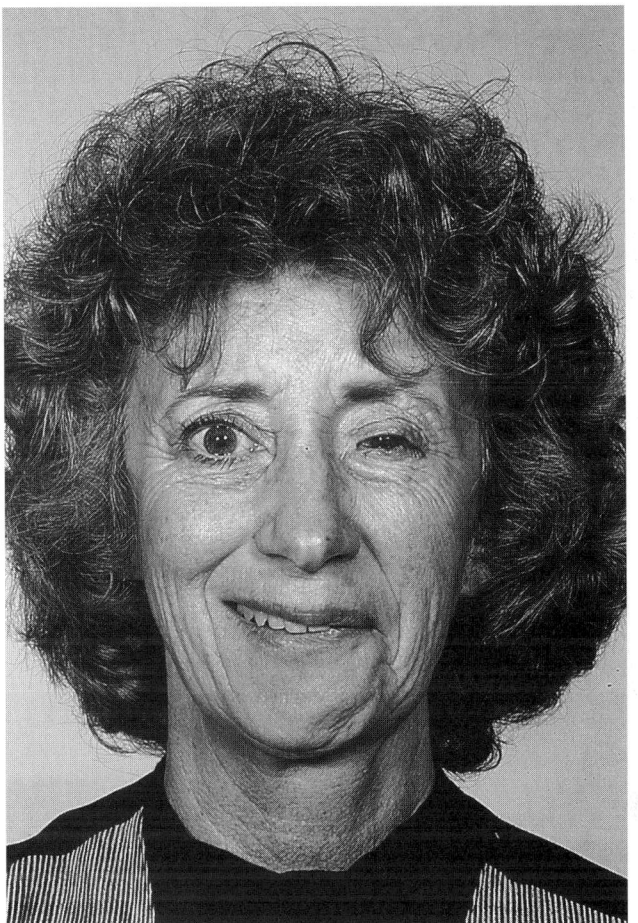

(c)

Fig. 52 (*Continued*) (c,d) I prefer a facio-accessory anastomosis when I cannot preserve the facial nerve. This patient's tumour is shown in Figure 13 (pp. 18–19) and it proved impossible to save the facial nerve in the medially arising acoustic neuroma. These photos were taken 9 months and 1 week after the anastomosis and show her smiling and whistling. She had trained herself to smile by tensing her shoulder girdle. I believe it is better to do this anastomosis than a facio-hypoglossal nerve anastomosis, which adds a tongue weakness to the facial weakness — insult to injury.

preserve the facial nerve much better if one obtains a good exposure of the nerve in the meatus rather than by passing dissectors blindly around the tumour towards the lateral-most extent of the meatus. Facial nerve monitoring I think is, on the whole, useful particularly when you first start operations for acoustic neuromas. I also find careful examination of the MRI scan

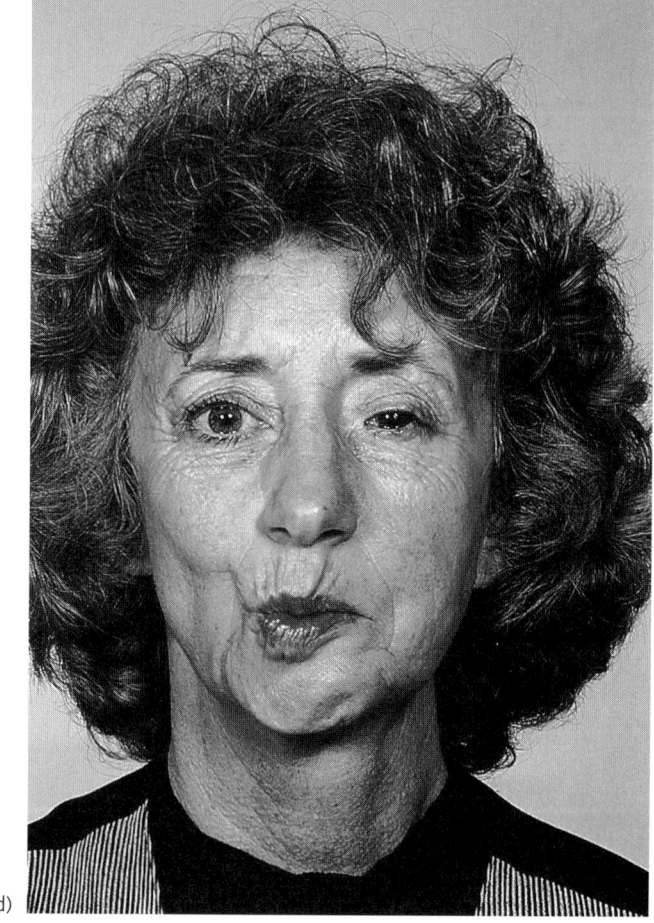

(d)

Fig. 52 (*Continued*)

allows an assessment of the relationship between the vestibule and semicircular canals and the meatus, which tells one how far laterally it is safe to drill
without damage to the inner ear (see illustrations in Chapter 2).

Having obtained sight of the two ends of the facial nerve I work around
the capsule of the tumour, mobilizing first one pole then the other, gradually
removing the tumour to make it smaller and smaller and easier to handle.
My only advice about how to preserve functional facial and cochlear nerves
is not to touch them! Touch the tumour, not the nerves and of course to preserve hearing one needs to preserve the internal auditory artery arising from
the anterior inferior cerebellar artery. If the nerve is stuck then sharp

dissection is better than blunt dissection which inevitably produces some traction injury to the nerve. If you find difficulty dissecting around in front of the capsule of the tumour, then you have to remove a wedge of capsule to reduce the bulk of the tumour. In this way you gradually make the tumour smaller, the last piece of tumour being attached to the seventh and cochlear nerves.

To reconstruct the internal auditory meatus I place a small piece of muscle in the depths of the meatus and then cover this with bone dust obtained from drilling the posterior fossa. Finally, I cover the dust with a layer of Surgicel. I have a low CSF leak rate through any opened air cells in the meatus using this technique.

It is important to close the dura in a watertight fashion (and this often demands an additional fascial graft taken from the occipital area) and to wax the exposed mastoid air cells well to prevent a CSF leak and rhinorrhoea. I routinely replace the craniectomy with removed bone as I believe this reduces the incidence of suboccipital pain, of which these patients sometimes complain. I did this first many years ago when I found I cured a patient's post-operative pain by performing a cranioplasty filling in the rather sunken defect remaining after a craniectomy to remove an acoustic neuroma.

The one thing that prolongs the patient's hospital stay is damage to the vagal group of nerves producing dysphagia. Therefore treat these nerves with the greatest respect! I always give these patients a 5-day course of antibiotics because the air cells are inevitably opened.

I should mention the position of the patient; the position I find the best I have not seen described in any literature but I can thoroughly recommend it. I place the patient supine and then 'recline' the patient so the head and upper body are 20° tilted up while the legs are also tilted 20° up. I then turn the head 90° to the opposite side (with a sand bag and bolster along the ipsilateral shoulder and chest) extending the head 20° to the trunk thus bringing the mastoid process horizontal. This position has two advantages over the simple supine position. First, the venous pressure is much reduced and second, the shoulder falls away naturally without the need to forcibly strap it away from the surgeon's view, which I think may obstruct the neck veins and increase the sigmoid sinus venous pressure. I use this position for all operations in the cerebello-pontine angle — try it!

What do you do if you cannot preserve the facial nerve? See Figures 13 (pp. 18–19) and 52(c). I prefer the facio-accessory anastomosis. Patients, with encouragement and determination, can learn to smile again. I tell them to practise in the mirror by tensing their shoulder girdle in order to smile. After a while it becomes second nature. I believe this is easier to do than 'tensing the tongue', and anyway it does not seem sensible to add a tongue weakness to a facial weakness by doing a facio-hypoglossal anastomosis.

Bilateral acoustic neuromas: neurofibromatosis Type II

I have commented already on my approach to these lesions under the general introduction of this chapter in the section 'how to preserve cranial nerves'. In fact I cannot guarantee to preserve hearing with these tumours; these are different, being multi-lobular and much more adherent to the cochlear nerve than unilateral acoustic neuromas. Neurofibromatosis Type II is indeed a frightful disease. These patients should only have an operation when their symptoms demand one. Do not operate on their scans; these will always show pathology of diverse nature.

Arteriovenous malformations

AVMs place great demands on the surgeon for two particular reasons. The first is the need for considerable judgement to decide on the best method of treatment, or indeed whether treatment of any sort is indicated. Secondly, they can be particularly challenging lesions to remove surgically. There are no miracles when dealing with these lesions. Walter Dandy once said that when faced with some AVMs you should tip your hat at them and walk on! Despite the advances the same is true today. It is all too easy for a young, or not so young, neurosurgeon to feel that he or she ought to tackle an AVM because a world-expert neurosurgeon would surely do the same. However expert and experienced the neurosurgeon, there are some AVMs that they would not tackle! Which ones do you tackle? It all depends on the natural history and this can, in part, be deduced by the mode of presentation. If an AVM has bled then the likelihood is that it will bleed again. If the AVM presents with epilepsy or a progressive neurological deficit due to ischaemia from 'steal', then the chances of bleeding in the future are less. Unfortunately it is less clear cut than this, for patients may have multiple small bleeds and be left with little functional deficit. On the other hand an AVM, and often a small AVM, may bleed catastrophically on the first occasion and kill the patient. It is well established that the risks of operation are greater if the AVM is large (more than 6 cm), if it is in an eloquent area (motor, speech or sensory cortex; internal capsule, basal ganglia or brain stem) or if there are deep draining veins, which usually mean deep supplying arteries. Thus, the risks of post-operative neurological damage have to be balanced against a risk of haemorrhage in the future. In general if the AVM is small and accessible it should be removed by operation. It becomes more difficult when there is a large lesion in or near an eloquent area and the lesion has not bled.

There are two other methods of treating AVMs: the first is by stereotactic radiosurgery (gamma knife or linear accelerator). This is suitable for lesions with a nidus of less than 2 cm diameter. How you measure the size of a nidus is, however, subjective and debatable. The main problem is that it may take 2–3 years for the radiation-induced endarteritis to obliterate the lesion. If the AVM has bled, then further bleeding may not be prevented in these early years and that of course is the aim of the treatment. Its use is more justified if the AVM has not bled and it is in an eloquent area. Radiosurgery is not, however, without complications, which are due to, usually (delayed) brain damage from radiation necrosis.

The second method is endovascular obliteration of the fistula or at least of the feeding arteries. In my experience this method does not eliminate AVMs. Nothing less than total elimination is satisfactory because a remaining fistula will open up again with time. However, this method is especially useful in conjunction with an operation. Thus, the endovascular method can obliterate significant feeding arteries and this is particularly useful if the deeper arterial input can be obliterated, as it is these arteries that are very difficult for the surgeon to deal with early in the operation. AVMs are often cone shaped with the base of the cone at the cortex and the apex of the cone leading down to the ventricle, with deep draining veins extending into the ventricle and deep feeding arteries from the choroidal vessels entering the AVM. The endovascular approach cannot unfortunately deal with the deep choroidal supply but by eliminating a lot of the inflow the surgeon's task is made much easier. The risk of NPBB bleeding is also reduced by carrying out pre-operative endovascular treatment, and reducing the high flow through the fistula.

I have one caveat concerning endovascular treatment. I have noticed that some vessels that appeared only 24 hours earlier to be completely obliterated by glue, at surgery have been seen to be recanalized with a cast of glue in the centre of the vessel lumen but with blood passing between the glue cast and the endothelium. This makes me a keen advocate of endovascular treatment as an adjunct to surgery but not as a long-term 'stand alone' solution for AVMs.

If the AVM presents with epilepsy then on balance surgical excision is more likely to stop the epilepsy than the trauma of the surgery to induce epilepsy. Thus, if the AVM is small (less than 6 cm) and in a non-eloquent area then surgery should be advised as the best chance of stopping the epilepsy as well as, of course, eliminating the risk of a future bleed.

How should the surgeon approach the difficult problem of whether to advise surgery? The general approach has been outlined in the chapter on judgement. The natural history as well as the clinical features need careful consideration. Experience and the availability of the various other methods of treatment also count. Angiography is an essential investigation but perhaps as essential, if not more essential, is an MRI scan. Never operate on an AVM without an MRI scan! It is immensely useful. The anatomy of the AVM in relation to the surrounding brain is best appreciated on the scan. The angiogram of course gives exact information about the arterial input but remember the draining veins are important for two reasons. First, the draining veins will lead the surgeon to the AVM once the flap has been turned, and secondly the surgeon needs to consider which draining vein, or veins, he or she is going to preserve until the end. Sometimes a single, large, tortuous draining vein can make life extremely difficult for the surgeon by obliterating the view of the anatomy of the AVM.

I spend a long time examining the angiogram and MRI scan so I build up a three-dimensional picture in my mind of the arteries, veins and nidal anatomy. One always needs to have a plan; in general it is to attack and eliminate the arterial input at the earliest stage. Once the red draining vein goes blue one knows the AVM has surrendered but never be tempted to make this judgement prematurely. Taking out the draining vein too early can make the AVM engorged, tense and extremely difficult to handle and then it starts pouring blood from all areas. I once had to carry out an emergency craniotomy for an AVM when the endovascular glue obstructed, not the fistula, but the draining vein. It was an operation that I shall remember although the patient did remarkably well considering the lesion was in the deep part of the dominate temporal lobe supplied by the posterior cerebral artery.

When removing an AVM the surgeon has to dance between dissecting too close to the AVM and risking haemorrhage from the lesion and being too far away, risking damage to the normal brain. The brain around the AVM has small vessels that are infuriatingly fragile and may be very difficult to coagulate. If they rupture they can retract into the surrounding brain and may be very difficult to find. Every AVM is different. Some are well defined and others are diffuse. Sometimes there are 'daughter' AVMs connected to the main AVM by a narrow isthmus. These can be dissected across, thus leaving the daughter AVM behind. This is the reason for routine post-operative angiography. I vary my plane of dissection according to how eloquent the brain is that I am dissecting. If a frontal lobe AVM is backing on to the motor cortex I will start my dissection anteriorly and leave a generous margin of brain around the AVM with the aim of eliminating the arterial input from the anterior and middle cerebral arterial branches, but as I dissect around the posterior extent of the AVM in the region of the motor cortex I dissect right up against the loops of the AVM.

The most feared complication after an otherwise successful operation for an AVM is NPBB. It must be admitted that this is sometimes, even often, an excuse for inadequate haemostasis or bleeding from a 'daughter' AVM left behind. Beware of placing Surgicel over a bleeding point, for this is not usually adequate. Before coming out, take away the Surgicel and have a good look around for bleeding points. If the AVM tapers down to the ventricle, put a pattie in the ventricle at the first opportunity to prevent blood filling the ventricles. This should be done whenever one operates inside the ventricles. If in doubt do an immediate post-operative CT scan rather than wait for clinical deterioration.

In my view there are two causes or subtypes of NPBB. I have always thought that the venous side of the AVM has been too much ignored. I had one patient with an AVM who presented with 'benign intracranial hyperten-sion' (severe papilloedema endangering eyesight) due to the high venous pressure in the superior sagittal sinus due to 'arterialized' blood being shunted directly into this sinus from a large adjacent AVM (Figure 53) This must often occur and profound alterations must exist to the normal cortical venous drainage to the superior sagittal sinus of both hemispheres when an AVM drains into the sagittal sinus. Just think what must happen when an

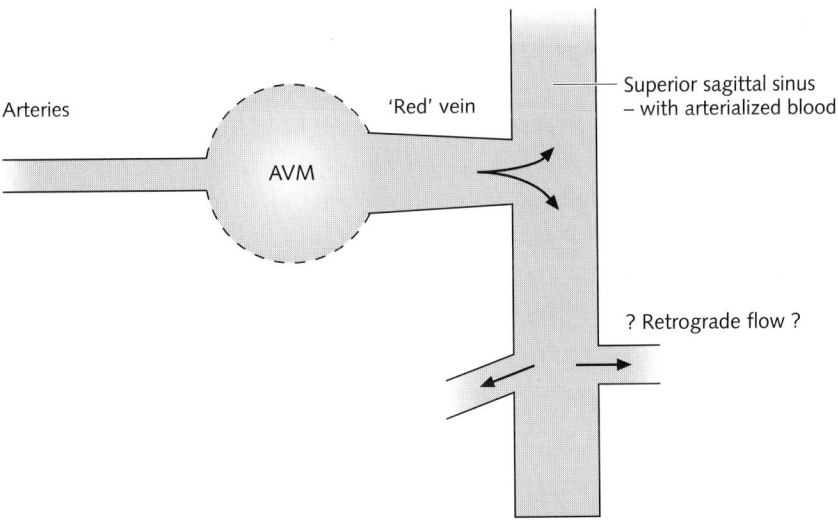

Fig. 53 Diagram highlighting the pressure changes in adjacent veins and venous sinus.

AVM shunt is suddenly eliminated. This high 'venous' pressure suddenly drops, and this must produce profound changes to the established but abnormal venous drainage that existed when the AVM was present. Little wonder I had one patient who developed severe swelling of the opposite hemisphere after removal of an AVM.

But 'arterial' NPBB does exist! For many years I doubted it until I had a patient with a large AVM. I removed it and congratulated myself that the lesion came out according to my pre-operative plan without hardly a drop of blood being spilt. About 2 hours post-operatively he deteriorated. I took him back to the theatre and there was generalized oozing. I tried excising more surrounding brain to find 'normal' non-bleeding brain but this was not a successful exercise. The only way to stop this bleeding was to hypotense the patient. Once this was done everything miraculously stopped bleeding. We kept him hypotensed for 48 hours in the intensive care unit and he made an excellent recovery. Remember the hypotension! If you come across this condition you will be pleased you did so. I do not propose to debate the various theories but it does seem to occur especially with high-volume, large-shunt AVMs and this is a good argument for trying to reduce the flow by pre-operative endovascular treatment. Indeed I regard the successful management of AVMs as a team effort between the endovascular and surgical therapists.

Flow aneurysms and arteriovenous aneurysms

Occasionally one sees an aneurysm on one of the feeding arteries. Sometimes, rarely in my experience, they bleed. Figure 54(b) shows an angiogram of such an aneurysm on a feeding artery to a thalamic/intraventricular arteriovenous malformation. This AVM could not be treated by endovascular methods and so I excised it surgically. The patient made a complete recovery and returned to his legal studies at Oxford University. Interestingly, the flow aneurysm disappeared on the post-operative angiogram. In general, therefore, remove the AVM and only worry about the aneurysm it if is still there after the AVM has been treated.

Trigeminal neuralgia

I do not propose to rehearse the arguments against the hypothesis of microvascular compression which I have published from time to time. I suppose these arguments are an exercise in 'skepticos'! Most surgeons would agree that there are times when a partial root section is indicated. I believe

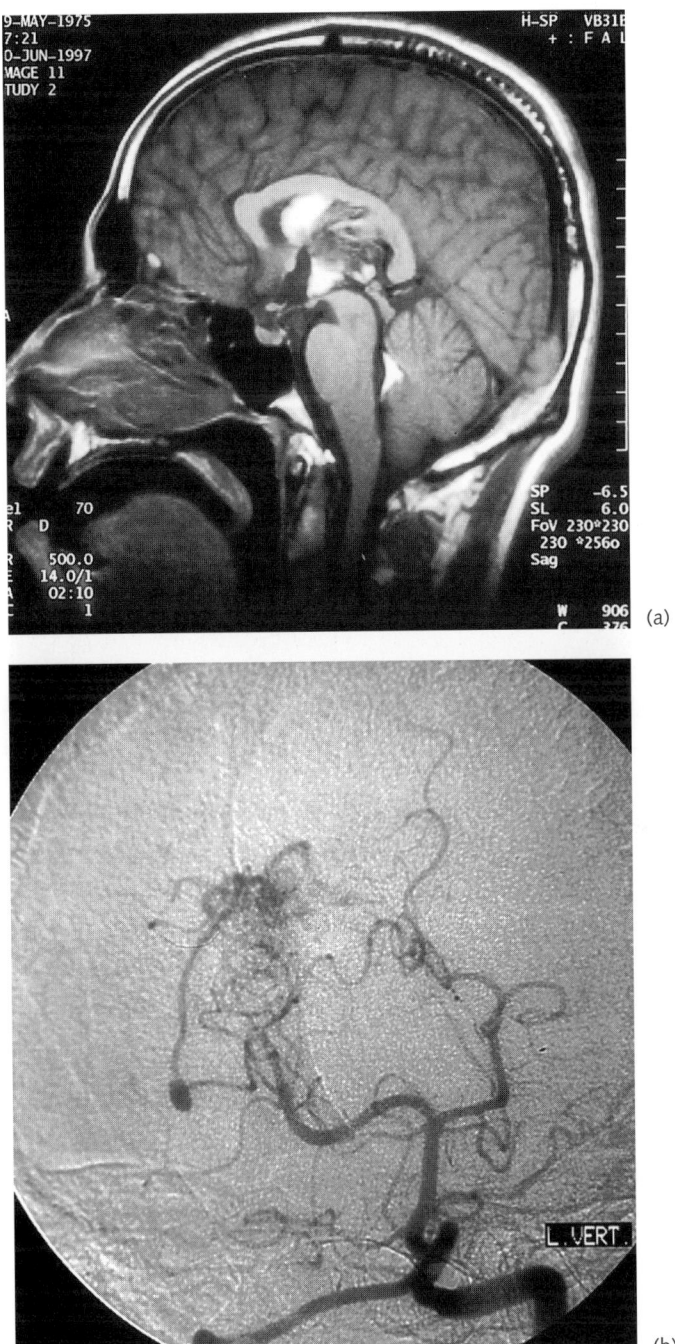

(a)

(b)

Fig. 54 (a,b) The AVM prior to operation. The MRI scan shows its position and the angiogram the lesion and the 'flow' aneurysm. (*Continued*)

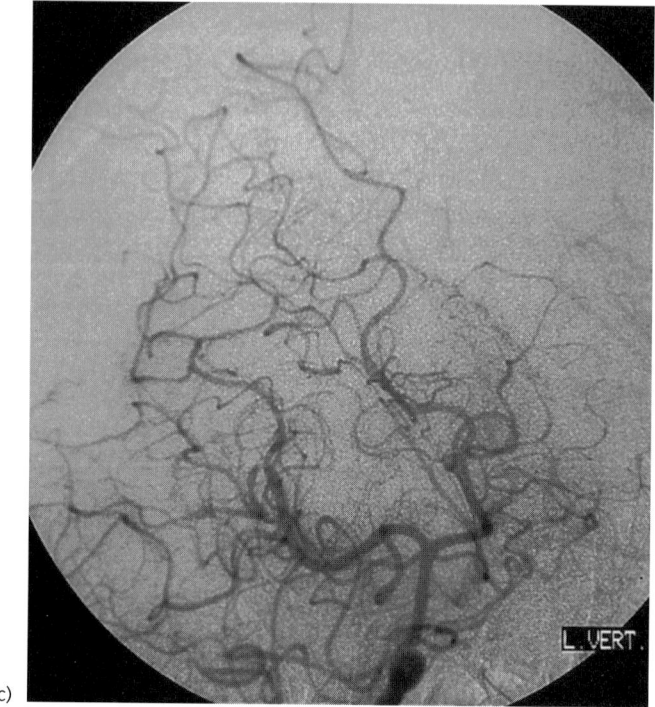

(c)

Fig. 54 (*Continued*) (c) The post-operative appearance after removal of the AVM. The flow aneurysm has disappeared.

the anatomy of the sensory root is less well appreciated than it ought to be, and is not described in standard texts. The three divisions are represented in the sensory root but as this rotates as it enters the brain stem, and because the degree of rotation varies from person to person, one cannot use external, fixed, anatomical markers to indicate these divisions. One has to use the motor root instead and Figure 55 indicates the relationship of the three divisions to the motor root. The first division occupies the pole of the sensory root immediately adjacent to the motor root, whereas the third division is at the opposite pole of the sensory root. I have found this works well: find the motor root (which is often double) and you will know where the sensory divisions are. This works 95% of the time for me.

Neurosurgical trainees do not always appreciate the distribution of the fifth nerve (which of course determines the distribution of trigeminal neural-

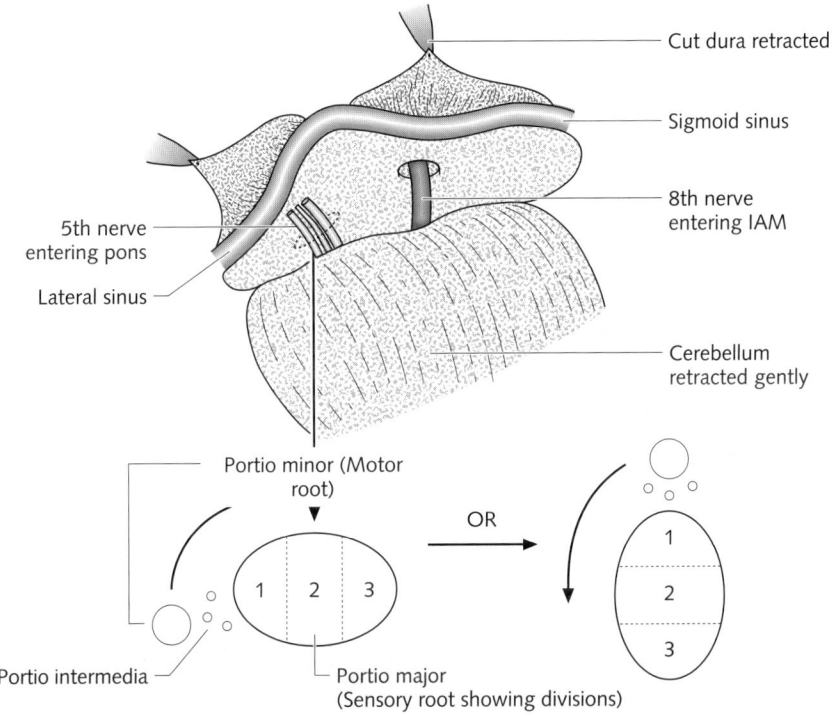

Fig. 55 How to find the divisions of the trigeminal sensory root. See text.

gia). Remember there are at least two or three finger widths of C2 opposite the angle of the mandible. In other words, the part where men shave adjacent to the angle of the mandible is C2. The trigeminal nerve does, however, supply the tragus, the anterior part of the external auditory meatus and the anterior superior part of the pinna (the amount varies). The posterior part of the external meatus is supplied by the seventh nerve. Neuralgia of the nervus intermedius does exist! Twenty years ago I had one patient, a doctor from Brazil, who had intense pain inside the external auditory meatus. The pain was exacerbated each time he inserted a stethoscope into his ears. So severe was the pain that he had become addicted to strong analgesics. I cut his nervus intermedius, a tiny cotton thread of a nerve, between the seventh and eighth nerves in the posterior fossa, and he was immediately and completely cured.

How to do a Burr hole for an Extradural Haematoma
C.B.T. Adams—Radcliffe Infirmary, Oxford

1. Introduction
Think of an extradural haematoma if the patient is drowsy and has a skull fracture. DO A CT SCAN

2. Indication for a burr hole
– Extradural haematoma showing on CT; patient's conscious level rapidly deteriorating with evidence of brain-stem compression – that is dilated, sluggish or fixed pupil or pupils
– Unless a burr hole is done the patient will die or be damaged: You and the patient have nothing to lose and everything to gain. An inelegant burr hole now will do much more good than an elegant operation one hour or more later

3. Incision
– Shave scalp if time
– No local anaesthetic is necessary usually
– 4 cm incision over clot as shown on CT (This is on the side of the dilated pupil or fracture or at the site of the blow) This is usually in the temporal region – just above the zygomatic arch—curved as shown so it can be enlarged

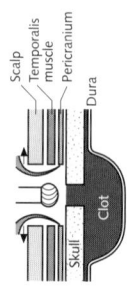

4. Incise right down to the bone. Do not stop to stop scalp bleeding

5. Scrape back pericranium
(periosteum) using periosteal elevator (or similar instrument) to expose skull
– Insert mastoid retractor – this will stop all the bleeding
– Leave the retractor in

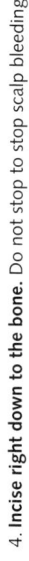

Retractor
Scalp
Temporalis muscle
Pericranium
Fracture
Skull
Dura

6. Perforate the bone using a perforator
Dark clot will ooze out
The dura (inner skull periosteum) will not be seen as it is stripped away by the blood clot. Do no more than **just** perforate the skull
This will create a conical hole

Scalp
Temporalis muscle
Pericranium
Dura
Skull
Clot

7. Enlarge the perforation using a burr
The burr will enlarge the hole so the hole is nearly cylindrical

8. Blood clot will immediately ooze out. Suck the clot away by applying a sucker to the burr hole but DO NOT INSERT SUCKER INTO THE CAVITY – that will cause more bleeding and might damage the brain

Scalp
Temporalis muscle
Pericranium
Dura
Skull
Clot

9. It is now safe to transfer the patient to Oxford.
Phone 01865 311188
NB. 1. Leave the scalp retractor in! We will return it
2. Leave in the endotracheal tube and leave a drip up
3. Send any blood that has been cross matched with the patient
4. Send the CT scans with the patient
5. Well done! It really is very easy to do a burr hole, isn't it?

Fig. 56 'Safari neurosurgery'. How to do a burr hole!

Safari neurosurgery

How to do a burr hole: extradural haematomas

It is with considerable reluctance that I include this, but it has been suggested that this book may find itself in parts of the world where neurosurgeons do not exist. I will be delighted if this turns out to be the case and so I reproduce here a poster, made to encourage orthopaedic surgeons (and other non-neurosurgeons) to do a burr hole to let out most of the extradural haematoma before sending the rapidly deteriorating patient on a 1-hour (or more) journey to Oxford (Figure 56).

Most hospitals have CT scanners to tell you if there is an extradural haematoma and where it is. If you do not have a scanner the golden rule is 'make the burr hole at the site of the blow or injury' because it is there that the dura is initially stripped away from the skull and this initiates the extradural bleeding.

I have written about head injures and more basic neurosurgery in the *Oxford Textbook of Surgery* (see Further reading).

The future

When I was young the operating microscope was the future of neurosurgery and how well it has served us. The computer will control the future and indeed the future is with us in the form of the operating arm system. This allows precise localization of say, a subcortical cavernous angioma and its atraumatic removal. Stereotactic localization using computer software and CT scanning will also achieve the same, but I suspect the major future advance will be stereotactic radiosurgery. If so, it will have profound implications for skull base surgery, acoustic neuroma and even pituitary surgery.

Au revoir

It is usual to read a factual book of neurosurgery and know nothing of the author. Of course, being sceptical you would, in your own mind, have worried about what you read and challenged it, and in so doing have wondered about the author. In writing this small notebook, I have deliberately excluded what I thought were generally well known facts and assumed the reader's familiarity with them. I have given you some information, several prejudices, and I hope something of the art and philosophy of neurosurgery. It is not possible to do this without exposing something of myself—warts and all. So although you may have got to know me a little, I fear that I probably know you not, but who knows, we may meet one day. Neurosurgery is a world-wide, but not too large community and that is one of the great pleasures and privileges of being a neurosurgeon. That is why I say *au revoir* and not goodbye.

Being a good neurosurgeon depends first on being a good doctor. What makes a good doctor? Kindness, empathy, conscientiousness, the ability to make sensible decisions and judgements, to inspire confidence in the patient and the desire to do your very best for that patient. Whatever technological wizardry you possess, never forget kindness and empathy. Without them you are lost and so are your patients.

Neurosurgery is a demanding mistress: although when young it is necessary to spend long hours, day and night, attending to her needs, you must also not lose sight of life beyond the strict confines of neurosurgery. To be a good doctor, you need to be a fairly well rounded person, and you certainly need a wise and sympathetic shoulder to rest a worried and anxious head on. Life is a journey for each of us, and during this journey we keep learning. A neurosurgical life is no different. I like to think that during one's journey one makes a ripple as a pebble falling into the still water of a lake. This ripple spreads ever more widely and interacts with other ripples, sometimes neutralizing them, but other times joining and adding and providing momentum and so spreading wider and wider. In this way, each person's spirit lives on, even after their death. May your ripples be good and strong and spread widely, as you pass through your neurosurgical life, treating patients and teaching the next generation of doctors and neurosurgeons.

Further reading

I apologize for the number of references to my papers: this does not mean they have any special virtues but merely because I have made some unsubstantiated statements in the text that can be followed up, should the reader desire.

Adams C.B.T. (1983) Hemispherectomy: a modification. *J. Neurol. Neurosurg. Psychiatry* **46**: 617–619.

Adams C.B.T. (1984) Vascular catastrophe following the Dandy McKenzie operation for spasmodic torticollis. *J. Neurol. Neurosurg. Psychiatry* **47**: 990–994.

Adams C.B.T. (1988) The management of pituitary tumours and postoperative visual deterioration. *Acta Neurochir (Wien)* **94**: 103–116.

Adams C.B.T. (1989) Microvascular compression: an alternative view and hypothesis. *J. Neurosurg.* **57**: 1–12.

Adams C.B.T. (1994) Section on Neurosurgery (pp. 2137–2191). In: *Oxford Textbook of Surgery.* Morris P.J., Malt R.A., eds. Oxford University Press, Oxford.

Adams C.B.T. Hemispherectomy. In: *Operative Surgery.* Black P., Kaye A., eds, in press. Churchill Livingstone.

Adams C.B.T., Logue V. (1971) Some functional effects of operation for spondylotic myelopathy. *Brain* **94**: 587–594.

Adams C.B.T., Fearnside M.R., O'Laoire S.A. (1978) An investigation with serial angiography into the evolution of cerebral arterial spasm following aneursym surgery. *J. Neurosurg.* **49**: 805–815.

Adams C.B.T., Loach A.B., O'Laoire S.A. (1976) Intracranial aneurysms: analysis of results of microneurosurgery. *Br. Med. J.* **2**: 607–609.

Apuzzo M.L.J. (1993) *Brain Surgery, Complication Avoidance and Management.* Churchill Livingstone.

Cusick J.F., Steiner R.E., Berns T. (1986) Total stabilisation of the cervical spine in patients with cervical spondylotic myelopathy. *Neurosurgery* **18**: 491–495.

Falconer M.A. (1971) Anterior temporal lobectomy for epilepsy. In: *Operative Surgery.* Rob C., Smith R., eds. Butterworths, London.

George B., Lot G. (1995) Anterolateral and posterolateral approaches to the foramen magnum: Technical description and experience from 97 cases. *Skull Base Surg.* **5**: 9–19.

Kaye A.H. (1991*) Essential Neurosurgery.* Churchill Livingstone.

Kerr R.S.C., Cadoux-Hudson T.A., Adams C.B.T. (1988) The value of accurate clinical assessment in the surgical management of the lumbar disc protrusion. *J. Neurol. Neurosurg. Psychiatry* **51**: 169–173.

Malis L.I. (1990) The petrosal approach. *Clin. Neurosurg.* **37**: 528–540.

Naidich T.P., Brightbill T.C. (1996) The pars marginalis: Part I. A 'bracket sign' for the central sulcus in axial place CT and MRIs. *Int. J. Neuroradiol.* **2**: 3–19.

Ojemann G., Ojemann J., Lettich E., Berger M. (1989) Cortical language localisation in left, dominant hemisphere. *J. Neurosurg.* **71**: 316–326.

Rengachary S.S., Wilkins R.H. (1994) *Principles of Neurosurgery*. Mosby-Wolfe.

Teddy P.J., Adams C.B.T., Briggs M., Jamons M.A., Kerr J.H. (1981) Extradural diamorphine in the control of pain following lumbar laminectomy. *J. Neurol. Neurosurg. Pyschiatry* **44**: 1074–1078.

Yasargil M.G. (1984) *Microneurosurgery* (in 4 volumes). George Thieme Verlag, Stuttgart.

Yasargil M.G., Teddy P.J., Roth P. (1985) Selective amygdalo-hippocampectomy. Operative anatomy and surgical technique. In: *Advances and Technical Standards in Neurosurgery*, Vol. 12. Edited by Symon L. Springer Verlag, New York.

Index

Note: page numbers in *italics* indicate figures; those in **bold** indicate tables